STANDARD NOMENCLATURE
OF ATHLETIC INJURIES

Sub

Donald L. Cooper, M.D.
Richard C. Schneider, M.D.
Kenneth S. Clarke, Ph.D., Secretary

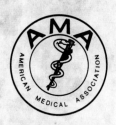

Single Copies to U.S., U.S. Possessions,
Canada, and Mexico, $1.50
Single Copies to all other countries, $1.75
Single Copies to Medical Students, Hospital
Interns and Residents, .75¢

OP-43-9801-Inv.-30E:368-10M
Printed in the U.S.A.

FOREWORD

Today's athletes are far superior to those of a generation ago, as has been demonstrated by the continuing advancement of records and more sophisticated performance in every field of sports. Improved health supervision of the athlete, along with better coaching and training methods, account for much of this advancement. Thus the "palm of victory" should be shared by team physicians and allied supervisory personnel who have combined to contribute to the development, prowess, and welfare of the athlete.

The Committee on the Medical Aspects of Sports of the American Medical Association and its Subcommittee on the Classification of Sports Injuries advocate the widest possible application of sports medicine for the athlete throughout the broadest range of participation—at every age, for both sexes, and from school to college on into the professional arena.

The value of health supervision of the athlete increasingly is recognized as no stronger than the connecting line: the medical record. Clear and factual documentation of the athlete's initial examination, participation, injury episodes, response to treatment, and succeeding studies are invaluable for continuing reference. Accordingly, sketchy or voluminous medical records colored with jargon, colloquialisms, and barbarisms are more misleading than helpful. The record must be presented in definitive language for uniform interpretation.

In recommending the appointment of its Subcommittee, the AMA Committee on the Medical Aspects of Sports recognized the importance of meaningful nomenclature for the reporting and tabulation of disabling conditions that occur in athletics. This recommendation eventuating in the publication of the *Standard Nomenclature of Athletic Injuries* (SNAI) provides a welcome contribution to medicine, as useful for physicians practicing internal medicine and surgery as for specialists involved in the study and care of athletes. The preface for the book by Alexius Rachun, M.D., chairman of the Subcommittee, reveals in detail its development. Features of the publication are striking; for example, there are precise definitions of terms commonly used in sports medicine, a cross-index to refer readers from supplementary or additional designations to preferred terms, and the committee's plan for updating the content in conformity with the most recent advances of modern medicine and surgery. Indeed, individual problems of nomenclature have been clarified, such as the mechanisms of sprains and strains, fractures, traumatic conditions of the vertebral column, and charleyhorse.

Invitations to attend the Subcommittee meetings were greatly appreciated by the staffs of AMA's *Current Medical Terminology* (CMT) and *Current Procedural Terminology* (CPT). The opportunity to observe the evolution and, subsequently, the completion of SNAI has been an interesting, stimulating, and rewarding experience. Particularly helpful was the opportunity to incorporate in CMT and CPT—which went to press during the early development of SNAI— significant data on the etiologies and/or effects of injuries due to athletic competition. Members of the Subcommittee on the Classification of Sports Injuries were most generous in sharing their knowledge and experience with the staffs of CMT and CPT at that time.

The value of SNAI to CMT thus illustrates well the increasing awareness that the lessons learned in sports medicine can benefit the total population. The application of sports medicine in general practice can be seen to depend partly on the observations and records derived from study and treatment of the athlete. The utilization of criteria gained from sports medicine for application in the study and management of noncompetitive individuals also is a significant contribution. Future editions of these publications will continue to reflect the contribution of sports medicine to medical practice as a whole.

Burgess L. Gordon, M.D., Editor
Current Medical Terminology
and
Current Procedural Terminology
AMERICAN MEDICAL ASSOCIATION

CONTENTS

PREFACE

The first meeting of the Subcommittee on Classification of Sports Injuries (Committee on the Medical Aspects of Sports) was held November 30, 1964. At that time, the Subcommittee discussed the charge given it by the AMA Board of Trustees: ". . . the development of a standard nomenclature relating to degree and type of injury in sports so that meaningful records and statistics concerning sports injuries and their cause and prevention can be maintained."

The establishment of the Subcommittee resulted from the recommendation of the parent Committee on the Medical Aspects of Sports. The Committee's review of existing athletic injury reports previously had revealed great variation in methods of recording and interpretation. Basic to this problem was the lack of a precise and uniformly understood medical terminology that adequately described the injuries and illnesses being experienced on the athletic scene. Where the interchange of such terms affects definitive diagnosis which in turn underlies appropriate treatment, valid reporting, reliable analysis, and consequent preventive measures, standardization of athletic injury nomenclature demanded high priority attention.

The American Medical Association since 1960 has endeavored to clarify problems of medical terminology as evidenced in its publication, *Current Medical Terminology* (CMT). While this progress in standardization greatly facilitated the Subcommittee's task, two factors posed unique problems for sports:

> 1) In no other area of medicine have nonmedical persons written so widely with respect to injury and disease. Familiarity of coaches, trainers, and physical educators with athletic injury causation and prevention is essential to the health supervision of the athlete. Yet, the variety of terminology and meanings presently found in current writing adds a sizable dimension to the perpetuation of ambiguous and misleading terms.
>
> 2) Certain injuries are peculiar to sports or gain clinical significance in the sports arena where explosive effort and violent contact take place and the motivation for earliest possible return to activity from injury is great. The physician who applies his medical skills in the athletic setting thus encounters diverse clinical problems from day to day. Each problem calls for immediate judgment, often without the benefit of previous experience or relevant discussion in a standard medical reference. There is more than a uniformity of terminology involved; there also must be an awareness that such injuries occur, have significance, and merit faithful recording.

Fundamental to an increasingly sophisticated health supervision of sports, therefore, is a common language that permits the sharing of accurate and complete information. One cannot agree or disagree with another if misinterpretation from a host of variable references is prevalent. Because of equivocal reporting, a recorded injury may misrepresent not only the degree of severity but also the true diagnosis; sometimes a significant condition may be overlooked because the index of suspicion is not sufficiently high. Such a situation is not conducive to constructive steps toward thorough understanding of specific athletic problems and preventive procedures.

It was these considerations that led the Subcommittee to set as its immediate goal the printing of this pilot publication. Each member accepted responsibility for reviewing AMA's CMT according to a particular anatomical assignment which involved selecting those terms appropriate for inclusion in an athletic nomenclature. Other athletic injuries or conditions that were not found in CMT but that merited inclusion also were added.

Concurrently, the Subcommittee surveyed the memberships of the National Athletic Trainers Association and the American College Health Association Section on Athletic Medicine for colloquialisms (and their respective definitions) used to depict medical entities of interest in sports. The response yielded over 150 such terms and substantiated the confusion that currently exists concerning even the most common terms. The survey also indicated a definite desire among trainers and team physicians for a clarifying reference.

At its fifth meeting (November 1965) the Subcommittee reviewed its progress during the year's period and agreed on the following:

- Sufficient concensus had been reached on preferred terms and their meanings to prepare the pilot pamphlet to be entitled *Standard Nomenclature of Athletic Injuries* (SNAI).
- Availability of SNAI prior to the 1966 football season would be advantageous for early feedback from its use.
- SNAI would be a compilation of medical entities described in a fashion to be pertinent to the recognition, diagnosis, recording, and reporting of conditions and injuries which occur in those sports normally conducted by schools and colleges.
- SNAI should serve as an instructional as well as functional reference for physicians, coaches, trainers, athletic directors, administrators, insurance groups, students, and others concerned with sports.
- Included in SNAI would be clinical conditions that are important in the preparticipation examination as well as injuries incurred from participation.
- SNAI would be based upon but not restricted entirely to CMT so that its terms could be related specifically to the athletic situation and the young age group involved with the objective of immediate clarification of current confusion.
- By subscribing to CMT's general format, SNAI would remain properly related to AMA's overall activities directed toward uniform terminology and lend itself to utilization in the next (4th) edition of CMT.

With the publication of SNAI, the Subcommittee's immediate responsibility has been met. To bring concensus and clarity out of disparity, however, is no short term goal but a continuous process of evaluation and revision. Changes and refinements in subsequent editions are to be expected.

The various innovations which received Committee concensus and met with consultant approval especially need the test of time and use in practice. Classification of sprains and strains by grade of severity should do much to reflect the relative functional seriousness of these common injuries. The precise classification of fractures should do much to reflect the mechanism of injury which must be understood in the quest for prevention. The classification of cerebral concussion by degree of symptom severity should do much to bring about careful recording of all head injuries that may be precursors to subsequent serious pathological events. The particular placement of a given sports vernacular— whether as a preferred term, additional term, glossary term, or exclusion— hopefully will be heeded by all who are sensitive to the Subcommittee's purposes.

Familiarization with SNAI perhaps is best accomplished by scanning the CROSS-INDEX to learn the scope and style of classification and then to become acquainted with the EXPLANATION OF SYMBOLS, the subcategories used to identify each term.

While the descriptive information relating to a term within these categories is meant to be representative of the entity, the reader can expect to find few cases that present all classical symptoms, signs, and other factors. Nonetheless, SNAI should be of assistance for differentiating one clinical entity from another, especially if differentiation has significance from either clinical or epidemiological perspectives. Where this purpose can be improved, we hope the reader will share his opinion with us.

Alexius Rachun, M.D., Chairman
Subcommittee on Classification of Sports Injuries
Committee on the Medical Aspects of Sports
AMERICAN MEDICAL ASSOCIATION

ACKNOWLEDGEMENTS

The Subcommittee is indebted to Fred V. Hein, Ph.D., Director, American Medical Association's Department of Health Education, for his assistance and guidance during the course of the project, and to Charles C. Edwards, M.D., Director, Division of Socio-Economic Activities, for his support with respect to both initiating and carrying out the project. Both the Subcommittee and the parent AMA Committee on the Medical Aspects of Sports are staffed administratively through the Division of Socio-Economic Activities and its Department of Health Education.

The Subcommittee also is grateful for the cooperation received from the Committee to Study Head Injury Nomenclature of the Congress of Neurological Surgeons. The neurological information designated in SNAI by an asterisk is based on that Committee's *Glossary of Head Injury Including Some Definitions of Injury of the Cervical Spine* (Williams & Wilkens Co., 1966).

Appreciation is extended as well to Donald H. O'Donoghue, M.D., whose personal comments and book, *Treatment of Injuries to Athletes* (W. B. Saunders Co., 1962), served as a key authoritative reference; Millard Kelly, physical therapist and head athletic trainer for the Detroit Lions professional football club, who served advantageously as the representative of the National Athletic Trainers Association for the Subcommittee project; and Donald Washburn D.D.S., Director, Bureau of Library and Indexing Service, American Dental Association, who provided the terms relating to dental-oral injuries with the assistance of Gerald J. Casey, D.D.S., Perry J. Sandell, M.P.H., and John E. Zur, D.D.S.

Meriting special thanks is Burgess L. Gordon, M.D., Editor of AMA's *Current Medical Terminology* (CMT), whose encouraging counsel supported and supplemented the Subcommittee's efforts. It is recommended that the reader of SNAI also obtain the more comprehensive CMT for coding information as well as overall nomenclature classification.

EXPLANATION OF SYMBOLS

PREFERRED TERM

at: Additional Term (synonym)

et: Etiology (the possible or actual causes of the disease or injury)

sm: Symptoms (the patient's complaints)

sg: Signs (physical findings revealed in the examination)

cm: Complications (the direct secondary process that *may* result from the the original condition)

lb: Laboratory data (such as that obtained from EKG or bacteriological culture)

xr: X-rays (radiographic findings)

pa: Pathology (tissue destruction or course of disease)

*   Based on information in:

> Congress of Neurological Surgeons Committee to Study Head Injury Nomenclature, *Glossary of Head Injury Including Some Definitions of Injury of the Cervical Spine*, Volume 12, Williams & Wilkins Co., Baltimore, 1966, 419 pp.

STANDARD NOMENCLATURE OF ATHLETIC INJURIES

Subcommittee on the Classification of Sports Injuries
Committee on the Medical Aspects of Sports

AMERICAN MEDICAL ASSOCIATION

ABRASION

at: Cinderburn; Floor Burn; Grass Burn; Mat Burn; Scrape; Skid Burn; Slide Burn; Strawberry
et: Friction; scraping of skin
sm: Local pain, stiffness; variable severity depending on size and site
sg: Tenderness; oozing; loss of epidermis; surrounding inflammation
cm: Infection, such as tetanus

ABSCESS

et: Pus-producing infection, usually staphylococcal; portal of entry: blister, callus, penetrating wound, laceration; communicable by contact
sm: Throbbing pain; malaise
sg: Tenderness; erythema; surrounding edema; fluctuation; fever; brawny swelling
cm: Suppurative lymphadenitis; septicemia
lb: Positive culture; leukocytosis

ABSCESS, AXILLARY

et: Infection, usually staphylococcal or streptococcal; portal of entry: axillary hair follicle; or, remote source via lymphatic route
sm: Pain on motion
sg: Bulging of axilla; erythema; tenderness; fever
cm: Septicemia
lb: Leukocytosis; positive culture

1

ABSCESS, PALMAR SPACE

- at: Collar Button Abscess; Web-Space Abscess
- et: Infection, usually staphylococcal; portal of entry: blister, callus, puncture wound, as in crew and gymnastics
- sm: Local pain; weakness of grip; perhaps malaise
- sg: Tendernesss, rapid swelling of palmar space, abscess pointing dorsally between metacarpals; indurated palm with loss of concavity; hand swollen dorsally; limited motion; pain elicited by extension of fingers; fever
- cm: Extension to adjoining tissue spaces, joints, tendon sheaths, and lymphatic vessels; osteomyelitis; contracture
- lb: Leukocytosis; positive culture

ACCESSORY TARSAL NAVICULAR FRACTURE

- at: Prehallux Fracture; Accessory Tarsal Scaphoid Fracture
- et: Forcible eversion with tight posterior tibial tendon
- sm: Pain over medial aspect of navicular
- sg: Tenderness sharply localized to medial aspect of navicular; pain elicited under forced passive eversion; undue prominence of medial aspect of navicular
- cm: Persistent disability
- xr: Accessory navicular avulsed from attachment

ACETABULUM FRACTURE

- et: Direct blow
- sm: Pain localized in hip, accentuated by motion; inability to bear weight; disability
- sg: Tenderness; muscle spasm about hip; laxity of tensor fascia lata; leg in position of external rotation
- xr: Fracture of acetabulum with or without displacement of femoral head

ACETABULUM FRACTURE, CHONDRAL

- et: Trauma as in fall from height
- sm: Local pain; inability to bear weight on limb; disability
- sg: Restricted motion of affected hip; crepitus; catch in hip
- cm: Persistent disability
- xr: May be negative or show irregular margin of acetabulum

ACHILLES TENDON STRAIN

- at: Pulled Heel Cord
- et: Forced dorsiflexion of ankle when calf muscles are contracted; vigorous exercise with muscular incoordination
- sm: Severe pain, especially on motion; disability
- sg: Grade by degree of severity: tender thickening over tendon about an inch above insertion; if complete rupture, defect palpable at musculotendinous junction; inability to walk on tiptoe; squeezing calf causes minimal or no plantarflexion; pain elicited on active plantarflexion or passive dorsiflexion
- cm: Persistent disability
- xr: May show soft-tissue defect in region of achilles tendon

ACHILLES TENDON TENOSYNOVITIS

- et: Excessive repetitive running or jumping; unaccustomed activity; wearing of tight shoes during activity
- sm: Local pain, especially on motion

sg: Tenderness and swelling over achilles tendon; crepitus; pain elicited on active plantarflexion and passive dorsiflexion
cm: Persistent disability

ACHILLOBURSITIS

at: Achilles Bursitis; Retrocalcaneal Bursitis; Superficial Calcaneal Bursitis
et: Excessive repetitive walking or running, especially in cleated athletic shoes; congenitally enlarged posterosuperior angle of calcaneus may be predisposing
sm: Pain localized usually proximal to insertion and anterior to tendon; disability
sg: May be confused with achilles tendon strain or tenosynovitis; active contraction of calf does not increase symptoms, while local pressure does; pain elicited by pressure in space anterior to achilles tendon or between skin and calcaneal tuberosity; retrocalcaneal bursitis rarely permits palpation of fluid but superficial calcaneal bursitis may show cystic mass
cm: Chronicity; calcific deposits in retrocalcaneal area
xr: Enlarged posterosuperior angle of calcaneus; calcific deposits if present

ACNE VULGARIS

at: Pimples; Blackheads
et: Hyperfunction of sebaceous glands; retention of sebum in orifices; endocrine factors; other unknown factors; onset usually in adolescence
sg: Numerous clinical types: comedo, papular, cystic, pustular, keloidal; distribution most commonly over face, neck, upper trunk; usually symmetrical
cm: Exacerbation; abscesses; pitted scars; secondary infection; psychic disturbance

ACROMIOCLAVICULAR SPRAIN, 1ST DEGREE

et: Fall onto point of shoulder; leverage force as in fall on adducted arm
sm: Local pain, especially on motion; some loss of shoulder function
sg: Tenderness localized over and behind joint; no deformity; slight swelling
pa: Incomplete tear of acromioclavicular ligament

ACROMIOCLAVICULAR SPRAIN, 2ND DEGREE

at: Acromioclavicular Separation
et: Fall onto point of shoulder; leverage force as in fall on adducted arm
sm: Local pain; moderate disability
sg: Prominence of joint; local tenderness; ligamentous and capsular laxity with increased mobility about joint
cm: Permanent deformity, disability; traumatic arthritis
xr: Outer end of clavicle displaced slightly upward and/or backward
pa: Tear of acromioclavicular ligament but not of coracoclavicular ligament

ACROMIOCLAVICULAR SPRAIN, 3RD DEGREE

at: Acromioclavicular Dislocation
et: Fall onto point of shoulder; leverage force as in fall on adducted arm

3

sm: Severe pain; marked disability
sg: Obvious deformity; local tenderness; ligamentous and capsular laxity with increased mobility about joint
cm: Permanent deformity, disability; traumatic arthritis
xr: Increased distance between clavicle and coracoid process; outer end of clavicle displaced upward and/or backward
pa: Complete tear of coracoclavicular and acromioclavicular ligaments

ADDUCTOR LONGUS STRAIN
et: Forced abduction of thigh
sm: Localized pain in ischiopubic region or upper medial aspect of thigh; disability
sg: Grade by degree of severity: ecchymosis; swelling; tenderness in ischiopubic region; pain elicited by passive abduction of thigh; tender firm mass more noticeable on active adduction against resistance; palpable defect between puboischium and muscle belly; bunching of muscle a short distance away from pelvis

ADDUCTOR MAGNUS STRAIN
et: Forced straddling injury; sudden violent muscular contraction as in running out of crouched position
sm: Acute pain in ischiopubic region which may radiate along medial aspect of thigh down to medial femoral condyle
sg: Grade by degree of severity: swelling; ecchymosis; tenderness localized along medial aspect of thigh with possible palpable defect in muscle belly; pain elicited by passive abduction and active adduction of thigh
xr: May show avulsion of bone fragment downwardly displaced from ischiopubic rami

ANAL FISSURE
et: Constipation as in dehydration for wrestling; infection; trauma; diarrhea
sm: Burning pain initiated by defecation
sg: Fissure usually in midline posteriorly; spasm of anal sphincter; bleeding
cm: Infection; disability; chronicity

*ANEURYSM, CEREBRAL
at: Berry Aneurysm
et: Congenital defect in muscle coat of cerebral arteries at angles of bifurcation of the vessels causing dilatation; subject to rupture upon constitutional stress
sm: Asymptomatic until ruptured; with onset of bleeding: at first, sudden severe headache, dizziness, vomiting, fainting, drowsiness, unconsciousness; later, painful stiff neck and backache
sg: Nuchal rigidity; semicoma; perhaps dilated pupils, drooping eyelid; paralysis of extremity; convulsions
cm: Subarachnoid hemorrhage; hemiplegia; aphasia; mental changes; death
lb: Lumbar puncture demonstrates bloody fluid, increased intraspinal and intracranial pressure
xr: Cerebral arteriography diagnostic; routine skull x-rays may show calcified aneurysmal wall, erosion of sella turcica

ANGIONEUROTIC EDEMA

at: Giant Urticaria; Circumscribed Angioedema

et: Allergy; infection; emotional distress; familial trait (rare); two to three days duration with successive attacks likely

sm: Nonhereditary type: transient sensation of distention in involved areas; no itching or pain. Hereditary type: abdominal pain; dysphagia; vomiting; dyspnea

sg: Single or multiple swellings; round, transitory, tense, nonpitting lesions; most commonly appears on face, mouth, hands, feet, genitalia; slight redness may be present; hereditary type includes edema of tongue, pharynx, larynx

cm: Obstruction of breathing caused by laryngeal edema (hereditary type)

ANKLE DISLOCATION, ANTERIOR

et: Excessive forcible dorsiflexion of foot; fall upon heel with foot in position of dorsiflexion

sm: Pain; disability

sg: Obvious deformity; heel shortened, forefoot lengthened, foot in position of dorsiflexion; distal ends of tibia and fibula are prominent behind; malleoli may remain in place or, if fractured, displaced with foot; generalized swelling and tenderness

cm: Traumatic arthritis; residual stiffness

xr: Anterior dislocation of ankle, usually accompanied by fracture of anterior margin of tibial articular surface; one or both malleoli may be avulsed

ANKLE DISLOCATION, POSTERIOR

et: Foot in plantarflexion with strong forward thrust applied to leg

sm: Pain; disability

sg: Obvious deformity; distal ends of tibia and fibula visible and palpable beneath skin over front of ankle; distance between anterior border of tibia and heel is increased markedly; inability to dorsiflex foot on leg; generalized swelling and tenderness

cm: Traumatic arthritis; residual stiffness

xr: Posterior dislocation of ankle, usually accompanied by fractures of one or both malleoli and/or posterior margin of tibia

ANKLE DISLOCATION, UPWARD

et: Compression trauma

sm: Pain; disability

sg: Obvious deformity; abnormal broadening of malleoli with approximation of heel to one or both malleoli; generalized tenderness and swelling

cm: Traumatic arthritis; residual stiffness

xr: Diastasis at inferior tibiofibular joint; talus pushed upward between tibia and fibula; usually considerable comminution of distal end of tibia and fracture of fibula

ANKLE EXOSTOSES, TALOTIBIAL

at: Osteochondral Ridges, Talotibial; Ankle Spurs

et: Direct trauma; repeated forceful impingement of talus on anterior margin of tibia, as in "drive" of athlete when cleats are fixed to ground

sm: May be asymptomatic; vague complaints of lost power; inability to run, cut, or jump at full speed without pain sg: Pinpoint tenderness directly over spur; forced dorsiflexion of foot elicits pain localized at anterior talotibial sulcus

cm: Avulsed spur producing loose body in ankle; traumatic arthritis

xr: Exostosis formation usually on back or front of tibia and/or back of head superiorly on talus; condition varies from simple change in contour to a spur of a centimeter or longer extending along whole width of bone

ANKLE FRACTURE, ABDUCTION, 1ST DEGREE

et: Foot forcibly abducted on leg

sm: Pain over medial malleolar region; moderate disability

sg: Localized tenderness and swelling over medial malleolus (swelling subsequently spreads); crepitus over medial malleolus; pain elicited by eversion of foot; no deformity

cm: Recurrent instability of ankle; nonunion of medial malleolus

xr: Fracture of medial malleolus, roughly transverse, at or just below inferior articular surface of tibia; little or no displacement of detached portion of medial malleolus

ANKLE FRACTURE, ABDUCTION, 2ND DEGREE

at: Includes Pott's Fracture; Dupuytren's Fracture; Bimalleolar Fracture; Trimalleolar Fracture; Cotton's Fracture

et: Foot forcibly abducted on leg

sm: Severe generalized pain; moderate to severe disability

sg: Obvious deformity with foot displaced laterally; generalized tenderness and swelling; pain elicited on inversion and eversion of foot; crepitus over medial malleolar and distal fibula regions; ankle mortise may have spring; limited motion of ankle

cm: Traumatic arthritis; malunion; prolonged disability

xr: Transverse fracture of medial malleolus at or just below inferior articular surface of tibia; fracture of distal end of fibula, transverse either above or below inferior tibiofibular articulation; or, diastasis of ankle with comminuted fracture of narrow portion of fibula 2 to 3" above joint and separation of a wedge-shaped fragment; also may have a posterior marginal fracture of tibia and displacement of foot; also may have avulsion of an intermediate fragment from tibia at points of attachment of inferior tibiofibular ligaments

ANKLE FRACTURE, ABDUCTION, 3RD DEGREE

at: Supramalleolar Fracture

et: Foot forcibly abducted on leg

sm: Severe pain; disability

sg: Obvious deformity, foot displaced laterally; generalized tenderness and swelling of ankle

cm: Traumatic arthritis; malunion; prolonged disability; residual stiffness

xr: Transverse fracture of lower portion of shaft of tibia plus fracture of lower fibula with diastasis of ankle joint

ANKLE FRACTURE, ADDUCTION, 1ST DEGREE

et: Foot forcibly adducted on leg

sm: Pain localized at lateral malleolus; moderate disability

sg: No deformity; swelling and tenderness localized over lateral malleolus; crepitus over lateral malleolus; pain elicited on passive inversion of foot

6

cm: Recurrent instability of ankle
xr: Transverse fracture of fibula at or below articular surface of tibia; little displacement

ANKLE FRACTURE, ADDUCTION, 2ND DEGREE

et: Foot forcibly adducted on leg
sm: Generalized pain; disability
sg: Obvious deformity; foot displaced inward; ecchymosis; generalized swelling and tenderness; crepitus
cm: Traumatic arthritis
xr: Transverse fracture of fibula at or below articular surface of tibia, plus fracture of medial malleolus beginning at or below inferior articular surface of tibia extending obliquely upward and inward to emerge on medial surface of medial malleolus; or, fracture of tibia may involve inferior articular surface with fracture line beginning at any point on that surface; or, tibial fracture line may begin at its lateral margin near tibiofibular joint and pass upward and inward to emerge on medial surface of shaft with entire inferior articular surface separated from bone and displaced upward and inward; or, medial malleolus or that portion of articular surface which is avulsed with it may be comminuted

ANKLE FRACTURE, ADDUCTION, 3RD DEGREE

et: Foot forcibly adducted on leg
sm: Severe pain, disability
sg: Obvious deformity; foot displaced inwardly; ecchymosis; generalized tenderness and swelling; crepitus
cm: Traumatic arthritis; malunion; prolonged disability; residual stiffness
xr: Fibula and tibia fractured transversely in their lower third and displaced medially

ANKLE FRACTURE, EXTERNAL ROTATION, 1ST DEGREE

at: Fibula Fracture, Distal Portion, Spiral or Oblique
et: Leg forcibly rotated inward with foot fixed on ground; foot forcibly rotated outward on fixed leg
sm: Pain localized at lateral malleolar region; moderate disability
sg: Slight deformity over lateral malleolus; possible crepitus; tenderness and swelling localized to lateral aspect of lower leg
xr: Fracture line begins at front of lateral malleolus just below inferior tibiofibular articulation and passes upward and backward across joint, emerging on posterior surface of fibula

ANKLE FRACTURE, EXTERNAL ROTATION, 2ND DEGREE

et: Leg forcibly rotated inward with foot fixed on ground; foot forcibly rotated outward on leg
sm: Pain becomes generalized but is most severe along lateral aspect of ankle; disability; inability to bear weight
sg: Obvious deformity; crepitus laterally, sometimes medially; general tenderness and swelling; may palpate defect below medial malleolus; possible spring to ankle mortise
xr: Fracture of distal fibula displaced outward as well as rotated outward; may be displaced backward; possibly accompanied by frac-

7

ture of posterior margin of tibia; may show diastasis at ankle joint or an avulsion of an intermediate fragment from lateral surface of tibia (rare)

ANKLE FRACTURE, EXTERNAL ROTATION, 3RD DEGREE

at: Distal Tibial Epiphysis Fracture-Dislocation
et: Leg forcibly rotated inward with foot fixed on ground; foot forcibly rotated outward on leg
sm: Generalized pain; severe disability
sg: Obvious deformity; foot displaced outward; generalized tenderness and swelling
cm: Malunion; growth deformity
xr: Fracture of distal fibula plus lateral displacement of distal tibial epiphysis or complete transverse fracture through distal tibia

ANKLE FRACTURE, LATERAL MALLEOLUS AVULSION

at: Chipped Ankle; Ankle Inversion Sprain-Fracture
et: Foot forcibly turned inward on leg while bearing weight upon it as in placing foot upon an uneven surface while walking or running
sm: Severe pain on outer side of ankle; disability
sg: No deformity; acute tenderness and possibly crepitus over area anterior to and below tip of lateral malleolus; marked swelling
cm: Recurrent instability of ankle in inversion
xr: Avulsion of tip of lateral malleolus; variable displacement medially and downward; inversion stress films may show increased talar tilt

ANKLE FRACTURE, MEDIAL MALLEOLUS AVULSION

at: Chipped Ankle; Ankle Eversion Sprain-Fracture
et: Foot turned forcibly outward on leg while bearing weight as in placing foot upon an uneven surface while walking or running
sm: Severe pain on inner side of ankle; disability
sg: No deformity; acute tenderness and possibly crepitus over medial malleolus; marked swelling
xr: Avulsion of tip of medial malleolus; variable displacement laterally and downward

ANKLE FRACTURE-SEPARATION, DISTAL TIBIOFIBULAR EPIPHYSES

et: Usually forcible abduction injury; may be of adduction type; occurs between ages 10-16
sm: Local pain; disability
sg: Obvious deformity; limited range of motion of ankle; generalized tenderness and swelling
cm: Growth deformity
xr: Epiphyses may be displaced in any direction but usually outward

ANKLE SPRAIN, DELTOID LIGAMENT

at: Ankle Sprain, Eversion; Ankle Sprain, Medial Collateral Ligament
et: Foot forcibly turned outward on leg while bearing weight as in placing foot upon an uneven surface while walking or running; fall from height
sm: Severe pain first felt on inner side and gradually spreads if severe

to entire foot and lower leg; inability to bear weight; disability
- sg: Grade by degree of severity: no deformity; swelling most marked anterior to and below medial malleolus, sometimes involving entire foot and lower leg; ecchymosis; acute tenderness over area anterior to and below medial malleolus sometimes extending around ankle joint and up leg; while abduction and eversion elicits pain, foot can be pressed directly upward against tibial articular surface without eliciting pain
- cm: Persistent instability of ankle
- xr: Undisplaced fracture of medial malleolus or avulsion of its tip ruled out by anteroposterior, lateral, and oblique views

ANKLE SPRAIN, FIBULAR COLLATERAL LIGAMENT

- at: Ankle Sprain, Inversion; Ankle Sprain, Lateral Collateral Ligament
- et: Foot forcibly turned inward on leg while bearing weight as in placing foot upon an uneven surface while walking or running; fall from height
- sm: Severe pain first on outer side, gradually spreading if severe to entire foot and lower leg; inability to bear weight on foot; disability
- sg: Grade by degree of severity: no deformity; swelling; ecchymosis; acute tenderness over area anterior to and below tip of lateral malleolus sometimes extending around ankle joint and up leg; while adduction and inversion elicits pain, foot can be pressed directly upward against tibial articular surface without eliciting pain
- cm: Persistent instability of ankle
- xr: Undisplaced fracture of lateral malleolus or avulsion of its tip ruled out by anteroposterior, lateral, and oblique films; in severe cases, inversion stress films may show increased talar tilt
- pa: Varying degrees of injury of capsule, anterior tibiofibular ligament, anterior talofibular ligament, calcaneofibular ligament, and posterior talofibular ligament

ANKLE SUBLUXATION, RECURRENT

- et: Foot forcibly inverted, rupturing anterior talofibular and calcaneofibular ligaments; incomplete healing of previous similar injury; spontaneous reduction
- sm: History of ankle sprains; variable pain and disability; insecurity and weakness upon weight bearing
- sg: With heel inverted and forefoot adducted, talus tilts outward and forward leaving a well-defined sulcus immediately in front of lateral malleolus in comparison with opposite ankle; variable tenderness and swelling.
- cm: Persistent disability
- xr: Inversion stress films show talus tilt as much as 20-25° in ankle mortise compared to opposite ankle

ANSERINE BURSITIS

- et: Repeated friction; external blow to region of pes anserinus
- sm: Sharp pain localized to upper anteromedial side of knee
- sg: Tenderness located at upper anteromedial side of knee under the unattached portion of the medial hamstring tendons; pain aggravated by flexion and extension of the knee; crepitus; occasionally swelling
- cm: Chronicity

9

ANTERIOR TIBIAL COMPARTMENT SYNDROME

at: Volkmann's Ischemia of Leg
et: Unaccustomed repetitive activity; direct trauma; localized infection
sm: Severe, chronic pain made more severe by function, not disappearing with rest
sg: Loss of function of anterior tibial and toe extensor muscles with ensuing foot drop; passive stretching of involved muscles produces red, glossy, and warm skin over area; marked tenderness and hardness of fascia over involved space; occasionally accompanied by peroneal nerve injury and consequent sensory loss over dorsum of foot, lateral side of lower leg
cm: Severe disability, if unrecognized early, due to ischemic necrosis and irreparable scarring
pa: Rapid swelling of muscle within anterior tibial compartment or hemorrhage into this space; edema, extravasation of red blood cells; replacement of muscles by fibrous scarring and inelastic non-contractile muscle groups

ANTERIOR TIBIAL TENDON TENOSYNOVITIS

et: Excessive repeated use of tendon; tendency of athlete to pronate heel so that talus rotates downward and inward in relation to foot while running; unaccustomed repetitive activity
sm: Pain localized to anteromedial aspect of foot at or near tendon insertion
sg: Tenderness, swelling, erythema localized along course of insertion of tendon; crepitus; pain elicited on active dorsiflexion or passive plantarflexion of foot
cm: Recurrence; persistent disability

ANXIETY REACTION

at: Conversion Reaction; Hysteria Neurosis; Anxiety State
et: Functional; psychogenic
sm: Acute or gradual onset of anxiety out of proportion to any apparent organic cause; feelings of inadequacy, fatigability, irritability, inability to concentrate, depression, urgency; dry mouth; nausea; vomiting; vertigo; giddiness; diarrhea; diplopia; other symptoms
sg: Nonspecific; dilated pupils; flushed face; hyperventilation; tachycardia; may have loss of gag and/or corneal reflexes

APOCRINITIS

et: Bacterial infection of single apocrine glands, often after use of deodorant, in association with intertrigo or secondary to dermatitis; surface microflora trapped within occluded apocrine glands at sites such as axillae, groin, and perianal area
sm: Local pain; disability
sg: Discrete tender masses deep in skin; erythema often absent
cm: Abscess formation

APPENDICITIS, ACUTE

et: Infection: most commonly of escherichia coli, enterococcus, beta hemolytic streptococcus; obstruction of lumen due to lymphoid hyperplasia, adhesions, fecaliths, foreign bodies, intestinal parasites
sm: Early: usually epigastric, hypogastric, or periumbilical pain. Later: pain localized in right lower quadrant; nausea; vomiting; early and persistent loss of appetite

sg: Tenderness in right lower quadrant; muscular guarding; rebound tenderness; diminution of peristalsis; fever; tachycardia
cm: Gangrene; perforation; peritonitis; liver abscess; subdiaphragmatic abscess; intestinal obstruction
lb: Leukocytosis

ARCH SPRAIN, STATIC

et: Constant stress of weight superimposed on arch; repetitive vigorous exercise with long hours on feet; occurs early in season often as a result of change from regular shoes with arch to flat athletic shoes
sm: Pain along arch promptly relieved by rest
sg: Tenderness along plantar ligament from attachment at the calcaneus to its attachment near the metatarsal heads; not limited to "flatfoot" individuals
cm: Persistent disability

ARCH SPRAIN, TRAUMATIC

et: Acute, violent overstretching of calcaneocuboid ligament, plantar ligament, longitudinal arch, lateral ligaments of foot, and/or inter-metatarsal ligaments; repeated episodes of overmotion; may be elicited from running in light shoes or barefooted
sm: Pain; difficulty in walking; inability to run
sg: Variable degree of severity; tenderness over involved area; possible swelling and ecchymosis
cm: Chronicity; persistent disability

ARTHRITIS, SUPPURATIVE

at: Pyogenic Arthritis; Purulent Arthritis; Septic Arthritis; Pyarthrosis
et: Pyogenic organism, usually blood-borne: staphylococcus, strepto-coccus, pneumococcus, gonococcus
sm: Chills; anorexia; malaise; prostration; acute pain in joint accentu-ated by movement
sg: Swollen, tender joint; erythema; brawny induration, thickening of periarticular tissue; fluctuation; muscular spasms limit movement; joint usually in position of flexion; fever; tachycardia
cm: Osteomyelitis; ankylosis; deformity
lb: Increase in white blood cells; aspiration demonstrates turbid fluid containing polymorphs, often with positive culture
xr: Decalcification; formation of new bone
pa: Purulent effusion; erosion of articular tissue

ARTHRITIS, TRAUMATIC

et: Repeated stress on joint articulating surfaces; contributing factors include irregularity of surfaces from previous injury or disease, loose bodies in joint, malalignment of joint from congenital or growth abnormalities
sm: Gradual onset with progressive increase in pain and restriction of movement
sg: Bony thickening about joint palpable; mild synovial effusion; no increased local warmth, synovial thickening, muscle spasm; vari-able degree of impaired joint motion; coarse crepitus palpable and/or audible on movement; deformity in late stages (usually past middle age)
cm: Severe disability
lb: Sedimentation rate not elevated; aspiration demonstrates clear, straw-colored fluid

11

xr: Spurring or lipping of joint margins from formation of osteophytes; serial films show progressive irregularities of joint margins; subchondral sclerosis; diminution of cartilage space; no rarefaction

ASTHMA, BRONCHIAL

et: Extrinsic: Response of susceptible bronchial tree to specific allergic or nonspecific irritative stimulus; most common external antigens include dusts, pollens, fungal spores, feathers, insecticides, lint; onset usually in first four decades of life. Intrinsic: usually secondary to infection of respiratory system; emotional disturbances, tension, physical exertion often contributory; possibly histamine reaction

sm: Dyspnea; sense of suffocation; pressure in chest; nonproductive cough; termination of paroxysmal attack marked by increased cough, expectoration of mucoid sputum

sg: Obvious respiratory distress; wheezing; prolonged expiration; coarse musical rales and squeaks

cm: Emphysema; chronic bronchitis; pneumonia

lb: Sputum demonstrates Curschmann spirals, Charcot-Leyden crystals, eosinophils

xr: Increased illumination of lung fields; low diaphragm with reduced motion during attack

ATHLETE'S FOOT

at: Tinea Pedis; Dermatophytosis; Foot Ringworm

et: Infection by Trichophyton, Candida albicans, Epidermophyton floccosum; host susceptibility involved; insidious onset

sm: Burning; itching; pain

sg: Multilocular vesicles, scaling, maceration, oozing, crusting, fissure between toes and on plantar surface of toes and feet

cm: Invasion of nails; secondary infection; dermatophytid reaction

BARTON FRACTURE

et: Fall onto outstretched hand

sm: Local pain; disability

sg: Wrist deformity; swelling; possibly crepitus

cm: Malunion; Sudeck's syndrome; permanent disability

xr: Marginal fracture of distal radius with fragment plus subluxation of carpus; fragment may be volar or dorsal

BASEBALL FINGER

at: Mallet Finger; Hammer Finger

et: Direct blow to tip of finger; extension of finger against firm resistance

sm: Local pain; disability; inability to extend distal phalanx

sg: Dropped finger tip; tenderness localized to dorsum of finger; bony fragment palpable if present

cm: Permanent flexion deformity of distal phalanx

xr: Negative unless bony fragment avulsed with tendon

pa: Avulsion of intrinsic phalangeal extensor at its insertion, with or without a portion of the bony tubercle attachment

BENNETT'S FRACTURE

et: Blow along axis or on dorsum of clenched thumb; striking with fist as in boxing

sm: Local pain; disability

12

sg: Deformity over proximal end of first metacarpal; swelling, tenderness, crepitus; increased motion at joint

cm: Traumatic arthritis; permanent disability; good reduction essential

xr: Fracture-dislocation of distal end of first metacarpal with fracture line extending into the metacarpal joint; large proximal fragment displaced upward and backward; small distal medial fragment remains in position; fracture may be incomplete with no displacement of fragment

BICIPITAL TENOSYNOVITIS

et: Unknown; trauma to anterior aspect of shoulder; irritation of tendon within bicipital groove; strain on biceps brachii musculotendon unit; repetitive hard throwing

sm: Local pain; disability on abduction and external rotation, and backward flexion and external rotation; stiffness

sg: Tenderness, crepitus on pressure over bicipital groove; tendon may be palpable if subluxated

cm: Chronicity; persistent disability; tendon rupture

BLISTER, FRICTION

et: Pressure and friction on a localized skin area; ill-fitting or stiff shoes; poorly applied adhesive tape

sm: Local pain; impaired movement; variable severity depending on site, size, and time of rupture

sg: Vesicle surrounded by reddened area; tenderness

cm: Infection; septicemia

BONE CYST, SOLITARY

et: Unknown; usually occurs in upper end of humerus before puberty, rarely in adults

sm: Usually asymptomatic until traumatized; discomfort, pain localized to area of involvement after light trauma, such as throwing a ball

sg: Possibly swelling if traumatized

cm: Pathological fracture

xr: Circular, translucent area of rarefaction in metaphysis, near epiphyseal line of humerus; cortex possibly thin, ballooned; may disappear spontaneously

pa: Lacunar absorption of bone by osteoclasts; solid fibrous tissue-mass or cystic cavity with aseptic fluid replacing space; hemorrhage with giant cells

BONE DEFECT, FIBROUS METAPHYSEAL

ct: Development defect, not true neoplasm; usually disappears after about two years from onset

sm: Usually asymptomatic

sg: None

cm: May form a fibroma which behaves like a tumor, i.e., a non-osteogenic fibroma; may predispose to pathological fracture

xr: Incidental finding; small bowl-shaped defects located eccentrically, usually in distal femoral metaphysis; bony margins are sclerotic and frequently scalloped but cortex is absent peripherally; ossification gradually occurs, resuming normal trabecular pattern

pa: Filled with fibrous tissue in chaotic pattern interspersed with varying amounts of foam cells and multinucleated giant cells

13

BONE FIBROMA, NONOSTEOGENIC

et: Temporary localized cessation of ossification; abnormal periosteal growth; developmental defect, not true neoplasm; long bones of lower limbs more frequently involved

sm: Pain localized over affected area especially on motion of contiguous joint; mild disability

sg: Swelling and tenderness localized over affected area, especially if traumatized

cm: Pathological fracture; malignant degeneration (rare)

xr: Defects may persist, grow, and eventually become central or at least involve a large area while remaining eccentric; marginal sclerosis and scalloping persist and become more marked; lesions develop a trabecular or locular appearance

pa: Cellular fibroma containing a varying number of multinucleated giant cells; clusters of macrophages containing lipids or iron frequently seen; less vascular than true giant cell tumors and more obviously fibroblastic; rarely multiple; vivid rusty color containing discrete bright yellow foci

BONE TUMOR, GIANT CELL

at: Osteoclastoma

et: Unknown

sm: Pain localized over affected area; disability

sg: Painful motion and stiffness of contiguous joint; local swelling gradually increasing, bony in texture; crepitant feeling

cm: Tends to recur after local removal; sometimes acts as frank malignant tumor metastasizing through blood stream to lungs; pathological fracture

xr: Destruction of bone substance, with expansion of cortex; tumor tends to grow eccentrically and often extends as far as articular end of the bone

pa: Bone trabeculae may remain within tumor giving it a faintly loculated appearance; consists of abundant oval or spindle-shaped stromal cells profusely interspersed with giant cells that may contain as many as 50 nuclei

BOUTONNIERRE DEFORMITY

at: Buttonhole Deformity

et: Trauma to dorsal aspect of middle phalanx of finger; excessive forcible flexion of proximal interphalangeal joint

sm: Local pain; disability

sg: Flexion deformity of proximal interphalangeal joint with inability of extension; local tenderness, swelling

xr: Negative unless bone fragment avulsed with tendon

pa: Avulsion of central portion of phalangeal extensor tendon at its insertion on the dorsal tubercle of the middle phalanx

BRACHIAL PLEXUS STRETCH INJURY

at: Brachial Plexus Traction Injury

et: Direct blow to the supraclavicular area with contralateral extension of the head and neck and posterior thrust of the involved shoulder

sm: Burning sensation, numbness, weakness; perhaps paralysis of ipsilateral arm, forearm, and/or hand

sg: May find complete areflexia and hypalgesia of the extremity or part of it with nondermatomal localization

14

lb: EMG important in ruling out ruptured cervical disc
xr: Cervical spine, clavicle, and shoulder views exclude osteoarthritic spurs or fractures; myelogram may show associated tear in cervical nerve root sleeve

*BRAIN SYNDROME, CHRONIC

at: Punch Drunk Syndrome; Chronic Cerebral Injury
et: Presumably, repeated head trauma as in boxing, leading to a form of chronic neurophysiological disorder characterized by emotional and/or mental impairment and/or motor deficit
sm: Mental confusion; tinnitus; giddiness, euphoria; personality changes
sg: Gradual and progressive onset; may be associated with confabulation, hallucinations, lack of associated movements, unsteadiness in gait, masked facial expression
lb: Lumbar puncture may show increase of protein content in cerebrospinal fluid
xr: Air study may show presence of increased sulci if air is in subarachnoid space; enlargement of ventricles suggests brain atrophy

BRONCHITIS, ACUTE

et: Bacterial or viral infection; allergic, chemical, or physical irritants
sm: Sore throat; hoarseness; cough; expectoration; malaise; chills
sg: Sibilant or sonorous ronchi; brassy persistent cough; occasional wheezing
cm: Chronic bronchitis; bronchopneumonia; bronchiectasis
lb: Leukocytosis; cultures of sputum may show etiology
xr: May have increased bronchial markings

BUNION

et: Congenital metatarsus primus varus; great toe persistently forced laterally by enclosure in tight stockings, narrow pointed shoes
sm: Pain; difficulty wearing footwear; disability
sg: Angular deformity at metatarsophalangeal joint; thick-walled bursa over medial prominence; local tenderness; skin over joint is hard and reddened; impaired joint motion
cm: Inflammation; suppuration; osteoarthritis
xr: Lateral angulation of great toe; periostitis and exostosis over medial aspect of metatarsal head

BURN, CHEMICAL

at: Lime Burn
et: Contact of skin with caustic chemicals such as lime, analgesic balm, other topical applications; allergic susceptibility of host may be contributory
sm: Pain; sensation of heat
sg: Erythema; swelling; tenderness; blistering; necrosis; sloughing
cm: Scarring; infection

BURN, 1ST DEGREE

et: Heat; wind; actinic rays of sun
sm: Warmth; pain
sg: Erythema; tenderness; stiffness; moderate edema

15

BURN, 2ND DEGREE

et: Heat; actinic rays of sun; therapeutic heat modalities
sm: Warmth; pain; frequently headache, malaise, nausea, vomiting
sg: Tenderness; erythematous vesicles; blebs; bullae; inflammation; fever; edema
cm: Infection

BURN, 3RD DEGREE

et: Heat
sm: Pain; malaise; nausea; vomiting
sg: Edema; necrosis; tenderness; possibly hypotension with shock
cm: Scarring; infection; gangrene; development of active duodenal ulcer
lb: Hypoproteinemia; anemia
pa: Destruction of epidermis, dermis, subcutaneous tissue, nerve endings

BURSITIS

ct: Trauma; attrition; chronic irritation
sm: Pain in region of bursa; varying disability
sg: Swelling, tenderness; palpable fibrinous or calcific granules in chronically inflamed superficial bursa; erythema
cm: Infection; adhesive capsulitis; stiffness; chronicity
xr: Calcific deposits if present
pa: Thickening of bursa wall; degeneration of epithelial lining; adhesions containing villi, calcific deposits

CALCANEAL APOPHYSIS AVULSION

et: Sudden violent strain on achilles tendon as in jumping; fall onto ball of foot
sm: Pain; inability to bear weight on foot; disability
sg: Swelling and tenderness around calcaneal tuberosity, posterior to malleoli on either side of achilles tendon; no swelling or tenderness in anterior portion of foot; separated fragment palpable in space between achilles tendon and posterior surface of tibia; pain elicited on plantarflexion of foot against resistance
xr: Separation of calcaneal apophysis from body of calcaneus

CALCANEAL APOPHYSITIS

at: Sever's Disease
et: Unknown; local trauma during adolescence
sm: Moderately disabling pain at posterior point of heel, usually somewhat below attachment of achilles tendon, especially on running or jumping
sg: Local tenderness; occasionally swelling; pain elicited by passive dorsiflexion of foot and active plantarflexion of foot
cm: May develop prominence of back of heel which is sensitive to pressure by heel of shoe
xr: Sclerosis of calcaneal apophysis frequently accompanied by fragmentation

CALCANEOCUBOID LIGAMENT SPRAIN

et: Excessive forcible inversion of foot

sm: Pain localized over lateral aspect of foot in calcaneocuboid region, especially on running; disability

sg: Tenderness and swelling over lateral aspect of foot in calcaneocuboid region; ecchymosis; pain elicited especially on active eversion and passive inversion of foot

xr: May show avulsion fracture of superolateral margin of cuboid with slight upward and lateral displacement of fragment

CALCANEUS FRACTURE, BODY

at: Os Calcis Fracture

et: Fall upon feet from a height, crushing and splitting of calcaneus by body weight being transmitted through talus

sm: Severe pain over heel; inability to bear weight; disability

sg: Swelling involving entire heel plus middle portion of foot and ankle; heel is broadened; definite bluish tint to tissues; long arch of foot flattened; eversion and inversion motion limited; excessive bone palpable behind and below lateral malleolus

cm: Prolonged disability; deformity; traumatic arthritis of subtalar joint or calcaneocuboid joint

xr: Variable: simple crack in bone without displacement to severe crushing with severe comminution and distortion of outline; lateral view shows depression of Boehler's angle; posteroanterior view shows lateral deviation and vertical splits

CALCANEUS FRACTURE, MARGIN AVULSION

et: Forced plantarflexion of foot

sm: Local pain; disability

sg: Tenderness and swelling localized over lateral aspect of foot near calcaneocuboid joint; pain elicited on plantarflexion and forced eversion of foot

cm: Persistent disability

xr: Fracture of overhanging anterosuperior margin of calcaneus at calcaneocuboid joint

CALCANEUS FRACTURE, SUSTENTACULUM TALI

et: Forced inversion of foot

sm: Sharp pain on inner side of foot; moderate disability

sg: Motions at ankle are relatively asymptomatic and unimpaired; variable amount of swelling over inner surface of calcaneus; acute tenderness just below tip of medial malleolus; calcaneus appears to be slightly displaced outward; foot tends to be held in pronation

cm: Painful flatfoot

xr: Compression or avulsion fracture of sustentaculum tali seen best by diagonal view through inner side of foot

CALCANEUS FRACTURE, TUBEROSITY AVULSION

et: Sudden violent strain on achilles tendon as in fall upon ball of foot or from muscular action as in jumping

sm: Pain; inability to bear weight; disability

sg: Swelling and tenderness around calcaneal tuberosity and posterior to malleoli on either side of achilles tendon; no swelling or tenderness in anterior portion of foot; separated fragment palpable in space between achilles tendon and posterior surface of tibia; pain

17

elicited by plantarflexion of foot against resistance

xr: Portion of calcaneal tuberosity avulsed and displaced upward; fracture line coincides closely with apophyseal line; or, superior portion may be avulsed; fragment may vary from small sliver beneath achilles tendon to a large mass comprising posterior portion of tuberosity

CALF STRAIN

at: Gastrocnemius, Soleus Strain
et: Sudden violent stress as in body weight forcibly throwing foot into extreme dorsiflexion; excessive forcible use in poorly conditioned person
sm: Severe pain deep in muscle especially on dorsiflexion of foot; disability
sg: Grade by degree of severity: inability to walk on tip-toe; defect may be palpable; swelling, edema, tenderness localized; ecchymosis; muscle spasm; diffuse inflammation; active contraction elicits bunching instead of flattening
cm: Prone to recurrence; thrombophlebitis; prolonged disability
pa: Can occur from origin to attachment of gastrocnemius and/or soleus usually in muscle belly; and frequently at musculotendinous junction between gastrocnemius and conjoined soleus tendon

CALLUS

at: Callosity
et: Repetitive friction; pressure on particular area
sg: Superficial, circumscribed horny patch of epidermis; flat, thick, dense, insensitive lesions; usually found on hands or feet
cm: Irritation; infection of subjacent tissues; lymphangitis

CARBUNCLE

et: Staphylococcal infection, usually of hair follicles and deep surrounding tissue; communicable by direct or indirect contact as in contaminated mats and towels
sm: Local pain; chills; malaise
sg: Fever; dusky red, hot, tense, tender, shiny area of skin covered with multiple pustular sinuses; ragged crater in center of lesion
cm: Lymphangitis; lymphadenitis; septicemia; distant abscess through hematogenous route
lb: Leukocytosis; positive culture of pus
pa: Multiple adjacent draining sinuses with central focus undergoing necrosis by liquefaction

CARPAL NAVICULAR FRACTURE

at: Scaphoid Fracture
et: Trauma indirectly transmitted upward from hand, usually due to fall onto pronated hand
sm: Pain on radial side of wrist; disability
sg: Acute tenderness over anatomical snuff box; swelling of wrist; limitation of wrist motion in dorsiflexion and radial deviation; weakness of grip
cm: Nonunion; traumatic arthritis
xr: Initial films may be negative; fracture line may be demonstrated after two weeks; often misdiagnosed as sprain; may require view with wrist dorsiflexed or in oblique position or with wrist against film with hand deviated to ulnar side

CARPOMETACARPAL, FIRST, DISLOCATION

at: Dislocated Thumb
et: Sudden violence forcing metacarpal upward and backward as in striking with fist
sm: Local pain; disability
sg: Local swelling; deformity at base of first metacarpal in region of anatomical snuff box; thumb shortened, held in moderate adduction; tenderness
cm: Chronicity
xr: Dorsal displacement of first metacarpal bone at carpometacarpal joint

CARPOMETACARPAL SUBLUXATION

et: Excessive forcible motion of wrist in any direction; spontaneous reduction
sm: Local pain; disability
sg: Tenderness on pressure over area; swelling; abnormal mobility
cm: Chronic abnormal motion, weakness

*CAUDA EQUINA CONCUSSION

et: Direct blow to base of spine
sm: Clinical syndrome characterized by immediate and transient impairment of neural function; numbness, weakness, or paralysis of several or all lower extremity movements; bladder and bowel impairment
sg: Transient with recovery: paresis, paralysis, and hypotonia of lower extremities; absence of patellar and ankle reflexes; saddle hypesthesia; loss of various dermatomes of lower extremities
xr: Myelogram negative
pa: Transient neurophysiological interruption

*CAUDA EQUINA CONTUSION

et: Direct blow to base of spine
sm: Pain radiating from injury site; numbness or weakness in lower extremities; bladder and bowel dysfunction
sg: Partial or permanent impairment of neural function; paresis; paralysis and hypotonia of lower extremities with hyporeflexia or areflexia; partial or complete dermatomal loss in lower extremities
pa: Structural alteration of axis cylinder; characterized by extravasation of blood cells and tissue necrosis with edema

CELIAC PLEXUS SYNDROME

at: Solar Plexus Syndrome; Abdominal Knockout
et: Direct trauma to abdomen in epigastric area over celiac plexus ganglion; thought to be a reflex dilatation of splanchnic blood vessels with consequent pooling of blood in abdominal vessels and lessened circulating blood volume to head
sm: Inability to take breath; fainting may occur; local pain
sg: Pallor; temporary respiratory dysfunction; sometimes unconsciousness

CELLULITIS

at: Phlegmon
et: Diffuse, spreading, edematous suppurative inflammation in soft tissue usually from streptococcal or staphylococcal infection; necro-

19

sis of subcutaneous tissue occasionally with small abscesses; may result from squeezed acne lesion or as wound complication
- sm: Local pain; chills; malaise
- sg: Erythema; edema; tender red area with flaring poorly defined borders; fever; lymphadenitis; lymphangitis
- cm: Uncontrolled spread; septicemia
- lb: Leukocytosis; positive culture

*CEREBRAL CONCUSSION, ACUTE, 1ST DEGREE

- at: Mild Cerebral Concussion
- et: Direct blow to head or helmet producing clinical syndrome characterized by immediate and transient impairment of neural function
- sm: No loss of consciousness; variable symptoms of momentary mental confusion, transient or no memory loss, mild tinnitus, mild dizziness and usually no unsteadiness
- sg: Perhaps none; or, appearance of brief period of mental confusion
- cm: Insidious cerebral hemorrhage; vulnerability to subsequent head trauma; post-concussion syndrome; perhaps post-traumatic epilepsy
- lb: EEG information helpful only if pretrauma EEG is available and post-trauma serial EEG's follow

*CEREBRAL CONCUSSION, ACUTE, 2ND DEGREE

- at: Moderate Cerebral Concussion
- ct: Direct blow to head or helmet producing clinical syndrome characterized by immediate and transient (*under five minutes*) impairment of neural function
- sm: Transitory loss of consciousness with brief but very definite retrograde amnesia; slight mental confusion, moderate tinnitus, moderate dizziness, moderate unsteadiness
- sg: Appearance of transitory unconscious state and subsequent mental confusion
- cm: Insidious cerebral hemorrhage; vulnerability to subsequent head trauma; post-concussion syndrome; perhaps post-traumatic epilepsy
- lb: EEG information helpful only if pretrauma EEG is available and post-trauma serial EEG's follow

*CEREBRAL CONCUSSION, ACUTE, 3RD DEGREE

- at: Severe Cerebral Concussion
- et: Direct blow to head or helmet producing clinical syndrome characterized by immediate and protracted (*over five minutes*) impairment of neural function
- sm: Prolonged unconsciousness, retrograde amnesia, mental confusion; severe tinnitus, dizziness; marked unsteadiness; general recovery rate very slow
- sg: Appearance of prolonged unconscious state and subsequent mental confusion
- cm: Insidious cerebral hemorrhage; vulnerability to subsequent head trauma; post-concussion syndrome; perhaps post-traumatic epilepsy
- lb: EEG information helpful only if pretrauma EEG is available and post-trauma serial EEG's follow

*CEREBRAL HEMORRHAGE, SUBARACHNOID

- et: Blow to head or helmet; ruptured cerebral aneurysm, arteriovenous anomaly; laceration of cerebral substance
- sm: Sudden severe head pain; dizziness; drowsiness; nausea, vomiting; stiff neck; photophobia; irritability; convulsion
- sg: Unconsciousness or semiconsciousness; delirium; nuchal rigidity;

positive Kernig's sign; bilateral pyramidal tract signs; possibly
hemiparesis or hemiplegia
cm: Recurrent hemorrhage; death
lb: Bloody or xanthochromic cerebrospinal fluid; increased cerebrospinal fluid pressure
xr: Angiography may demonstrate aneurysm, arteriovenous anomaly,
or presence of expanding lesion such as subdural or extradural
hematoma

*CEREBRAL HYDROMA, SUBDURAL

at: Subdural Cerebral Hygroma
et: Blow to head or helmet
sm: Headache; nausea, vomiting; drowsiness; irrationality
sg: Increasing drowsiness, homolateral dilated pupil; possibly hemiparesis; bilateral pyramidal tract signs
cm: Gradually increasing intracranial pressure; death
lb: May have elevated protein in cerebrospinal fluid and increased
pressure
xr: Displaced calcified pineal gland; arteriography shows enlarged avascular space between cerebral vessels and skull

*CERVICAL SPINE SPRAIN

at: Jammed Neck; Neck Sprain
et: Forceful, abnormal range of motion of neck
sm: Variable degree of severity of pain, strength and function loss
sg: Tenderness on palpation over involved area; muscle spasm variable
with severity of ligamentous injury; motion limited
xr: Fracture and dislocation ruled out; may demonstrate loss of normal curve
pa: Variable injury to interspinous-supraspinous ligaments (flexion injury) or to longitudinal ligaments (extension injury)

CHARLEYHORSE

at: Quadriceps Contusion
et: Direct blow to anterior aspect of thigh, characterized by intra-
muscular bleeding
sm: Pain generalized over area especially on movement; disability
sg: Variable degree of severity; pain elicited on passive stretching of
quadriceps; diffuse, deep tenderness; spasm; forced flexion past 90°
causes distress, active extension of knee against resistance causes
minor discomfort; ecchymosis; hematoma formation; extensive
swelling may migrate downward to knee resembling traumatic
synovitis of knee
cm: Traumatic myositis ossificans
xr: Initially, soft tissue swelling adjacent to cortex of bone; subsequently, possible calcification of soft tissue mass

CHONDROSARCOMA

et: Unknown; malignant tumor arises from cartilage cells and tends
to maintain its cartilaginous character; may develop in interior of
bone (central chondrosarcoma) or upon its surface (peripheral
chondrosarcoma); may arise without preexisting lesion or from
transformation of preexisting enchondroma
sm: Pain over affected part; varying disability
sg: Progressive swelling and enlargement of affected part; local tenderness

xr: Central type may burst through cortex whereas peripheral type shows as soft-tissue shadow growing outward from surface of bone; both types characteristically show blotchy areas of calcification within tumor mass

pa: May be highly cellular; cartilage cell nuclei tend to be swollen and double nuclei may be seen; much of tissue may appear relatively benign

CLAVICLE FRACTURE, INNER THIRD

et: Direct blow to sternal portion of clavicle
sm: Local pain; disability
sg: Little or no deformity; swelling; tenderness; crepitus
xr: Fracture of proximal third of clavicle

CLAVICLE FRACTURE, MIDDLE THIRD

et: Fall onto shoulder or outstretched arm
sm: Local pain; disability
sg: Local tenderness, swelling; deformity; crepitus
cm: Permanent deformity; injury to brachial plexus, pleura, blood vessels; nonunion
xr: Children: usually incomplete fracture or with overriding fragments; Adults: usually complete with downward, forward, and inward displacement of distal fragment

CLAVICLE FRACTURE, OUTER THIRD, 1ST DEGREE

at: Neer Type I Fracture of Distal Clavicle
et: Excessive force upon point of shoulder, driving humerus and scapula downward
sm: Pain over distal clavicle; disability
sg: Tenderness; crepitus; swelling over distal clavicle; slight deformity
cm: Persistent disability
xr: Fracture of distal clavicle with little or no displacement

CLAVICLE FRACTURE, OUTER THIRD, 2ND DEGREE

at: Neer Type II Fracture of Distal Clavicle
et: Force upon point of shoulder, driving humerus and scapula downward
sm: Pain over distal clavicle; disability
sg: Local tenderness; crepitus; swelling over distal clavicle; obvious deformity
cm: Nonunion; persistent disability
xr: Fracture of distal clavicle with proximal fragment riding above distal fragment
pa: Fracture plus coracoclavicular ligament rupture

COCCYGODYNIA

et: Direct blow as from fall; may appear insidiously without known cause
sm: Constant pain over coccyx
sg: Local acute tenderness
cm: Chronicity
xr: May reveal old displacement of coccyx; new fracture ruled out

COCCYX FRACTURE

at: Fractured Tailbone
et: Direct blow such as fall on buttocks
sm: Local pain; disability
sg: Tenderness; swelling; ecchymosis; rectal exam may elicit false motion or click; displacement palpable
cm: May lead to coccygodynia
xr: Fracture of coccyx with or without displacement

COLLES FRACTURE

at: Wrist Hyperextension Fracture
et: Indirect trauma, usually a fall onto outstretched pronated hand
sm: Local pain; numbness in fingers; limited supination-pronation
sg: Local swelling; ecchymosis; "silver fork" deformity with radial shortening; tenderness on palpation over distal radius
cm: Injury of median nerve; variable loss of function of hand, wrist; malunion; Sudeck's syndrome; permanent deformity
xr: Impaction of distal fragment of radius into proximal fragment dorsally, with radial shortening; loss of volar angulation; crushing of cancellous bone

CONTUSION

at: Bruise
et: Direct trauma causing tissue damage
sm: Local pain; stiffness; disability varies with site and extent
sg: Tenderness; ecchymosis; hematoma formation
cm: Traumatic myositis ossificans; calcification of damaged tissue mass

*CONUS MEDULLARIS CONCUSSION

et: Direct blow to spine
sm: Clinical syndrome characterized by immediate and transient impairment of neural function; interruption of bladder and bowel function; numbness of saddle area and portion of lower extremities
sg: Transient with recovery; hypalgesia over sacral area; paresis, hyporeflexia, and hypesthesia of lower extremities
xr: Myelogram negative
pa: Transient neurophysiological interruption

*CONUS MEDULLARIS CONTUSION

et: Direct blow to spine with structural alteration of spinal cord characterized by extravasation of blood cells and tissue necrosis with edema
sm: Numbness over the buttocks with bladder and bowel dysfunction; later, spastic gait
sg: Partial or permanent impairment of neural function; lower extremity and sacral hypesthesia or hypalgesia; weakness, spasticity, hyperreflexia of lower extremities
lb: Cerebrospinal fluid may demonstrate blood cells or elevated protein; jugular vein compression test may demonstrate partial block
xr: May show associated fracture; myelogram may show partial or complete block

CORN, HARD

at: Clavus Durum; Heloma Durum
et: Repetitive pressure and friction over particular area as from ill-fitted or poorly constructed shoes or small stockings; flexion-adduction deformity of toe (hammer toe) contributory
sm: Local pain; disability
sg: Redness, inflammation of lesion on dorsum of toe; thickening to overgrowth of soft tissue; sharp line of demarcation between corn and normal tissue
cm: Ulceration

CORN, SOFT

at: Clavus Molle; Heloma Molle
et: Repetitive pressure, friction of toe against toe from ill-fitted or poorly constructed shoe or small stockings
sm: Pain between toes, usually 4th to 5th; slight disability
sg: Circumscribed overgrowth between toes at bases of proximal phalanges; tissues yellowish if dry, white if macerated

COSTOCHONDRAL SPRAIN

et: Direct blow to costochondral joint or costal cartilage; compression of thorax; forcible torsion of trunk; may have subluxation or dislocation at joint with spontaneous reduction (displacement may persist)
sm: Mild to severe pain, aggravated on forceful expansion of chest or trunk motion; disability
sg: Grade by degree of severity: tenderness at costochondral junction or at costal cartilage; crepitus; slipping rib may be palpable; deformity variable with severity of sprain
cm: Chronic subluxation or dislocation
xr: Fracture ruled out
pa: Variable degree of injury to costochondral ligamentous-cartilaginous complex; fracture of costal cartilage may be associated

COSTOVERTEBRAL SPRAIN

et: Direct blow to rib; compression of thorax; torsion of trunk
sm: Pain in interscapular area, radiating anteriorly around chest on side of injury, aggravated on deep inspiration or rotation of chest
sg: Tenderness at costovertebral junction

*CRANIOCEREBRAL HEMATOMA, EPIDURAL

at: Extradural Cerebral Hemorrhage
et: Head trauma producing ruptured middle meningeal artery or torn dural sinus; may occur with or without skull fracture at middle meningeal groove in temporal region or at lambdoidal suture or lateral sinus in the occipital region
sm: Usually but not always loss of consciousness; injury may be followed by a period of mental clarity, usually of hours, rarely of days; relapse, loss of consciousness; possibly contralateral paresis or paralysis
sg: Possible scalp contusion; ipsilateral pupillary dilatation with bilateral pyramidal tract signs (tentorial or temporal lobe pressure cone); possible contralateral hemiparesis; slow pulse, rising blood pressure

cm: Death, especially if hematoma not decompressed immediately
xr: Skull films may show linear fracture of temporal bone or occipital bone

*CRANIOCEREBRAL HEMATOMA, SUBDURAL
at: Subdural Cerebral Hemorrhage
et: Head trauma producing tear of bridging cerebral vessels at vertex of skull where they enter the superior sagittal sinus or at base of skull
sm: Acute: headache; nausea, vomiting; irritability; diplopia; paralysis of contralateral extremities; coma; rapid progression.
Chronic: slow progression; intermittent headache; mental confusion with waxing and waning of consciousness; convulsion; hemiparesis; diplopia
sg: Acute: semicomatose to unconscious; unequal pupils; bilateral pyramidal tract signs; hemiparesis or hemiplegia possible.
Chronic: variable states of consciousness; memory loss, mental confusion; possible ipsilateral pupil dilatation; contralateral hemiplegia; bilateral pyramidal tract signs
cm: Death: increasing intracranial pressure; herniation of temporal lobe into tentorial incisura; herniation of cerebellar tonsilla into foramen magnum
lb: Acute: uncomplicated except for potential increased intracranial pressure; Chronic: EEG and/or brain scan may demonstrate abnormality

CRYPTORCHISM
at: Undescended Testis; Cryptorchidism
et: Congenital; probably associated with endocrine disorder, testicular dysgenesis
sm: Psychic disturbance
sg: Usually unilateral; testis not palpable in scrotum; three types: abdominal, retroperitoneal, inguinal; inguinal most common
cm: Associated hernia; sterility if bilateral

CUBOID FRACTURE
et: Direct trauma; severe crushing of foot; severe torsion injury
sm: Local pain; disability
sg: No deformity; local swelling and tenderness
cm: Traumatic arthritis
xr: Fracture of cuboid demonstrated

CUNEIFORM FRACTURE
et: Direct trauma; severe crushing of foot; severe torsion injury
sm: Local pain; disability
sg: May or may not have deformity; local swelling and tenderness
cm: Traumatic arthritis
xr: Fracture of first, second, and/or third cuneiform bone demonstrated

DENTAL CARIES
at: Tooth Cavity
et: Oral acidogenic bacteria; fermentable carbohydrates; other indefinite factors
sm: Local pain
sg: Chalky or dark area in tooth; carious lesion; destruction of tooth

25

cm: Pulpitis; osteitis; dental abscess
xr: Involvement of pulp; periapical abscess
pa: Progressive decalcified enamel; necrotic dentin

DERMATITIS, CONTACT
at: Dermatitis Venenata
et: Contact of skin with irritants such as tape, tincture of benzoin compound, penicillin, mercury applications, and other substances
sm: Variable degree of pruritus, burning pain
sg: Acute type: exposed portions of skin first affected with consequent edema, erythema, vesicles, bullae; rupture of vesicles, bullae, producing denudation, oozing, crusting, scaling. Subacute type: papules; thickening of skin; excoriations; crusting. Chronic type: lichenification; dryness; hyperpigmentation; fissures.
cm: Secondary infection with systemic manifestations; chronicity
lb: Patch test usually positive for suspected allergen

DERMATITIS, SEBORRHEIC
at: Seborrheic Eczema; Seborrhea Corporis
et: Unknown; associated with oily type of skin; constitutional diathesis; usually appears first on scalp, spreading to forehead, ears, face, brows, and other body areas; often associated with acne, rosacea, diabetes; psychosomatic factors
sm: Pruritus
sg: Scaling oily patches with indistinct margins and slight to moderate erythema at base; characterized by remissions and exacerbations
cm: Infection; blepharitis; otitis externa

DERMATOPHYTID
et: Sensitivity reaction to distant focus of dermatophytosis; manifested usually by lesions on fingers and hands
sm: Pruritus
sg: Round, vesicular lesions usually of fingers and hands; follicular, eczematous, erythematous lesions
cm: Recurrences
lb: Positive trichophytin skin test

DIABETES MELLITUS
at: Sugar Diabetes
et: Unknown; absolute or relative deficiency of insulin causing defective carbohydrate metabolism; hereditary predisposition; obesity frequently a precursor; aggravated by infection, trauma, surgery
sm: Variable if any at onset; unexplained weight loss, weakness; excessive thirst; polyuria; polyphagia
sg: Progressive emaciation with fine wrinkling of skin; other manifestations related to complications
cm: Insulin reaction; coma; susceptibility to infection, especially furunculosis; acidosis; peripheral neuritis; prolonged healing time; other late complications; complications usually avoided with proper control
lb: Glycosuria; ketonuria; elevated blood sugar; abnormal glucose tolerance test; diet and medication adjusted for level of exercise

*DISC RUPTURE, CERVICAL
at: Ruptured Cervical Intervertebral Disc; Ruptured Nucleus Pulposus; Protruded Disc (if displacement is from intervertebral space but not through the posterior longitudinal ligament, a condition which

26

may regress spontaneously); Herniated Disc (if fragment extrudes from interspace and through posterior longitudinal ligament, indicating complete recovery not likely)

et: Blow to head along longitudinal axis as in spearing; lifting, straining, twisting, with mechanical disadvantage

sm: Pain in neck, arm, and/or fingers, especially on tilting head backward or to involved side; accentuation of pain on coughing, sneezing, or straining; may have weakness in upper extremity; bladder or bowel impairment (rare)

sg: Pain radiating to neck, shoulder, arm, forearm, or hand elicited by percussion of neck or downward thrust on the head; may have loss of biceps or triceps reflex; if midline disc with cord compression, possibly tetraparesis or tetraplegia with complete sensory loss and hyperreflexia and hypertonia with pyramidal tract signs

cm: Compression of nerve root ("pinched nerve") with paralysis of specific muscles of upper extremity; possibly compression of spinal cord with paresis, paralysis of extremities and bladder, bowel incontinence and sensory loss to level of lesion

lb: Protein in cerebrospinal fluid may be elevated; EMG may be positive for nerve root damage after three weeks of compression

xr: Cervical spine films may show narrowed disc space; myelogram usually shows defect at involved interspace

*DISC RUPTURE, LUMBAR

at: Ruptured Lumbar Intervertebral Disc; Ruptured Nucleus Púlposus; Protruded Disc (if displacement is from intervertebral space but not through the posterior longitudinal ligament, a condition which may regress spontaneously); Herniated Disc (if fragment extrudes from interspace and posterior longitudinal ligament, indicating complete recovery not likely)

et: Trauma; lifting, straining, twisting with mechanical disadvantage; often no apparent cause

sm: Pain in back and/or in sciatic distribution, especially on bending to side of lesion; pain accentuated by coughing, sneezing, or straining; may have numbness in calf or foot, weakness in muscles of toe, foot on dorsiflexion; possible quadriceps weakness

sg: Limitation of motion; pain elicited by foot dorsiflexion with knee extended; tilt of spine away from side of lesion; positive straight leg raising test; may have sensory loss in lumbosacral dermatomes; may have loss or diminution of achilles or patellar reflexes; weakness in foot dorsiflexion

cm: Compression of nerve root with intractable pain, foot drop, bladder-bowel incontinence

lb: EMG possibly positive after three weeks of pressure; cerebrospinal fluid protein may be elevated

xr: May show narrowed interspace on plain x-ray film; myelogram usually positive for herniated disc

DROWNING, FRESH WATER

et: Submersion of head with ingestion of water; glottic spasm, followed by anoxia; relaxation of glottis with gasping aspiration of water into lungs; ventricular fibrillation; death

sm: Suffocation; unconsciousness

sg: Cyanosis; apnea; cardiac arrest; submersion for long period of time results in severe postmortem decomposition

lb: Potentially fatal disease or evidence of presubmersion trauma ruled out; low specific gravity of left heart blood; aquatic debris in lungs and/or stomach; diatomes in systemic circulation

pa: Water passes rapidly into blood stream across alveolar membrane in pulmonary bed producing profound hemodilution; ventricular fibrillation ensues due to either potassium intoxication or myocardial hypoxia

DRUG ERUPTIONS

at: Dermatitis Medicamentosa
et: Reactions due to ingestion, injection, inhalation, inunction of drugs reaching circulatory system; possible allergic influence; basic toxicity; normal pharmacodynamic action
sm: Variable: pruritus; malaise
sg: Lesions simulate practically every known cutaneous disease; eruption may be trivial and evanescent or severe and protracted; purpuric, exfoliative; disappearance with discontinuance of drug
lb: Skin tests are of limited value and dangerous

DYSMENORRHEA, PRIMARY

at: Painful Menstruation; Essential Dysmenorrhea
et: Unknown; psychogenic factors; congenital anomalies; systemic diseases
sm: Cramplike lower abdominal pain, most severe during first days of menstruation; weakness; nausea; vomiting; cold sweating; fainting; onset at or shortly after menarche; occurrence on ovulatory cycles
sg: Pallor; vague, diffuse tenderness over lower abdomen; menstrual clots may be present

DYSMENORRHEA, SECONDARY

at: Acquired Dysmenorrhea
et: (1) Tubo-ovarian inflammatory disease. (2) External endometriosis. (3) Mechanical obstruction of cervix, displacement of uterus; pelvic tumors, especially submucosal fibroids
sm: (1) Pain through entire cycle, becoming more intense at time of menstruation; possibly irregular bleeding. (2) Pain at onset of menstruation, subsequently reducing in intensity; dyspareunia. (3) Cramping pain during menstruation
sg: (1) Uterus adherent; irregular, soft tubo-ovarian mass. (2) Nodules in posterior cul-de-sac; rigidity, tenderness of uterosacral ligaments. (3) Dark blood; leukorrhea; stricture of cervix with evidence of past infection or surgery

EAR, CAULIFLOWER

at: Ear, Traumatic Deformity; Prizefighter's Ear; Wrestler's Ear
et: Repeated friction, contusion of auricle; subsequent formation of scar tissue
sm: Usually asymptomatic; sensitivity to cold; psychic disturbance
sg: Enlargement, wrinkling, puffiness, firmness of auricle

EAR DRUM, TRAUMATIC PERFORATION

et: Direct blow to external ear; direct tear of drum from instrument
sm: Pain; tinnitus; diminished hearing
sg: Visible perforation; bleeding
cm: Infection; loss of hearing; chronic otitis media

EAR, HEMATOMA, ACUTE

at: Early Cauliflower Ear
et: Contusion, repeated friction of auricle, as in wrestling and boxing, characterized by intra-auricular hemorrhage and edema

sm: Moderate to severe pain
sg: Swelling; discoloration; local fluctuation
cm: Deformity (cauliflower ear) if untreated; infection may occur after aspiration (rare)
pa: Small hematoma beneath perichondrium on anterior aspect of ear; blood changes to serous fluid within a week if unaspirated

EAR, IMPACTED CERUMEN
at: Wax in Ear
et: Excessive secretion of wax in external auditory canal; eczema; constitutional predisposition
sm: Sensation of fullness or obstruction in external ear; intermittent impaired hearing; tinnitus; possibly pain
sg: Dry, hard, impacted cerumen visible; lateralization of sound to obstructed ear
cm: Otitis externa

EAR, OTITIS EXTERNA, ACUTE
at: External Ear Dermatitis; Swimmer's Ear
et: Bacterial infection; allergy; swimming in contaminated water; loss of local natural resistance to infection from prolonged and repeated swimming
sm: Burning pruritus; acute pain; tinnitus; impaired hearing
sg: Hyperemia of auditory canal; gray or brown secretion in canal; fever; pain elicited by traction on tragus
cm: Chronicity
lb: Positive culture; fungus often present but not pathogenic

EAR, OTITIS MEDIA, ACUTE
et: Respiratory infections; obstruction of eustachian tube; rapid descent in airflight; lymphoid hyperplasia; allergies
sm: Earache; sensation of fullness, numbness in ear; autophony; headache; malaise
sg: Fever; red, bulging eardrum; landmarks obscured; usually loss of conductive type hearing
cm: Ruptured eardrum; mastoiditis; cavernous sinus thrombosis; meningitis; septicemia
lb: Exudate from paracentesis reveals positive culture; leukocytosis

ELBOW DISLOCATION, ANTERIOR
et: Direct blow to point of flexed elbow as in a fall
sm: Severe pain; disability
sg: Elbow fixed in near-complete extension; rounded condyles of humerus palpable at point of elbow; olecranon is absent from normal position; local swelling, tenderness
cm: Nerve, vascular injury; traumatic myositis ossificans; residual partial disability
xr: Olecranon rests on anterior surface of lower humerus; radial head is anterior to and above external humeral condyle

ELBOW DISLOCATION, POSTERIOR
et: Forcible hyperextension at elbow; fall onto outstretched hand with elbow extended and forearm supinated
sm: Severe pain; disability
sg: Elbow fixed in moderate flexion; increased anteroposterior diam-

eter of elbow; swelling; olecranon prominent and higher than normal; fullness in cubital fossa over front of elbow
cm: Injury to ulna, median, and radial nerve; vascular injury; traumatic myositis ossificans; associated fractures; residual partial disability
xr: Olecranon and head of radius displaced posteriorly with humerus distal to coranoid process

ELBOW OSTEOCHONDRITIS DISSECANS
et: Unknown; spontaneous ischemia; trauma involving capitellum or radial head
sm: Pain on movement; perhaps locking; limitation of extension movement
sg: Swelling, mild effusion; synovitis
cm: Traumatic arthritis
xr: Synovitis with distention of joint capsule; fragmentation of capitellum or radial head with widening and flattening of involved surface; loose bodies may be demonstrated

ENDOMETRIOSIS
at: Pelvic Endometriosis
et: Unknown; endometrial tissue transported from uterus to extrauterine site; endometrium developing in situ in ectopic location; direct extension from uterus
sm: Increasingly severe secondary dysmenorrhea; pain beginning just prior to menstruation, relieved shortly after onset; rectal pain accentuated by defecation, rectal or vaginal examination; dyspareunia; menorrhagia; irregular bleeding; cyclic rectal bleeding, hematuria coinciding with menstruation
sg: Small, tender fixed nodules in the uterosacral ligaments or rectovaginal septum; adherent ovarian cysts without evidence of external infection; decrease in mobility of pelvic structures; small, tender, bulging blue cysts in vagina with adherent mucosa; small mulberry-like cervical nodule resembling erosion

EPIDIDYMITIS, ACUTE
et: Nonspecific infection; mumps; trauma; reflux of urine in vas from excessive straining as in weight lifting; gonorrhea
sm: Pain in posterior scrotal and inguinal area; chills
sg: Swollen, tender epididymis; erythema, edema of scrotal skin; inflammatory reaction along spermatic cord; fever; spontaneous resolution unless complicated by abscess
cm: Abscess; orchitis; sterility; chronic epididymitis
lb: Leukocytosis

*EPILEPSY, FOCAL
et: Unknown; associated with acquired or congenital cerebral lesions; formerly used to designate seizures which begin with motor or somatosensory disturbances, but now includes other phenomena, e.g., a convulsion in which an odor precedes the attack is considered to be a seizure arising from a focus in the middle temporal region
sm: Variable, related to nature of seizure
sg: May be none if sensory in nature; if motor, signs limited to seizure of given area

cm: Development of grand mal seizures or status epilepticus
lb: EEG demonstrates dysrhythmia such as spike wave or spike focus from a given area of the brain cortex

*EPILEPSY, GRAND MAL

at: Major Epilepsy
et: Unknown; associated with acquired or congenital cerebral lesions; sudden, excessive, disorderly discharge of cerebral neurons
sm: Seizure characterized by loss of consciousness, tonic spasms of trunk and extremities followed in a few seconds or minutes by repetitive generalized clonic jerking, frothing at mouth, incontinence of bladder and/or bowel; may have preconvulsive aura of giddiness, apathy, headache, disagreeable taste or odor, nausea, yawning, depression, tingling and numbness in fingers or lips, flashes of light, muscular aching
sg: Unconsciousness; increased tonus in all four extremities initially, followed by flexion and extension of them; may have involuntary movement of eyes or head to one side, tongue biting, stertorous respirations, suspended respiration, cyanosis, frothy saliva, absent tendon and corneal reflexes
cm: Status epilepticus; fracture of lumbar spine
lb: EEG: Interictal—high voltage bursts of spike wave, spikes or slow waves; Ictal—sequence of abnormal discharges, series of rapid spikes or spike waves, polyspike waves; Postictal—flat or slow waves

*EPILEPSY, JACKSONIAN

et: Unknown; may be due to tumor, congenital condition, or scarring from traumatic lesion
sm: Progressive involvement
sg: Focal motor or sensory seizure which progresses by marches such as a seizure starting in the face with clonic movement followed by a spread to the arm with clonic movement and then to similar involvement of leg
lb: EEG usually demonstrates a spike and wave type of pattern starting at the site of the focal seizure and then spreading out over the cerebral cortex

*EPILEPSY, PETIT MAL

at: Pykno-Epilepsy; Minor Epilepsy
et: Relationship of trauma is controversial; possibly hereditary; acquired form associated with traumatic, infectious, neoplastic, vascular pathology of brain, drugs, and variety of general conditions or diseases
sm: Attacks of brief impairment of consciousness, seconds to minutes; often associated with flickering of the eyelids and mild twitching of mouth; amnesia
sg: Dazed appearance; staring, vacant expression; rhythmic motion of eyelids or head; pallor; incontinence. Astatic type: sudden loss of postural control
lb: EEG Interictal—brief bursts of diffuse spike waves or slow waves; Ictal—extended bursts of diffuse three per second spike waves

*EPILEPSY, POST-TRAUMATIC

at: Includes: Early Post-traumatic Epilepsy (if appearing a few weeks to one month post-trauma), a condition suggesting recurrent attacks unlikely; Late Post-traumatic Epilepsy (if appearing more than one month post-trauma), a condition suggesting recurrent

attacks likely
et: Head trauma
sm: Convulsive state with no pretraumatic history of convulsive manifestations; no other systemic or cerebral condition reasonably associated with convulsions
sg: Reasonable certainty of brain damage resulting from traumatic incident of magnitude; location of injury related to type of seizure
lb: EEG consistent with type of seizure demonstrated

*EPILEPSY, PSYCHOMOTOR
at: Temporal Lobe Epilepsy
et: Unknown; hereditary, congenital, or acquired cerebral lesions, usually in temporal lobe
sm: Attacks characterized clinically by impairment of consciousness
and amnesia for the episode; often associated with semipurposeful
movements of arms or legs and sometimes with psychic disturbances such as hallucinations, perceptual illusions, amnesic states
sg: Altered auditory, visual perception, partial consciousness, auto-
matic behavior; convulsions, chewing, smacking or licking lips,
tonic spasms of extremities; turning of head, eyes to one side
cm: Mental deterioration, rarely of severe degree
lb: EEG: Interictal—spikes or spike waves from temporal lobes, especially in sleep; ictal —spreading rhythmic sharp waves with onset
in temporal region; postictal—focal temporal slow waves

EPIPHYSEAL PLATE COMPRESSION FRACTURE
at: Epiphyseal Plate Injury, Type V
et: Severe crushing force through epiphysis to one area of epiphyseal
plate; occurs in joints moving in one axis, such as ankle; occurs
before epiphysis closure in growing children
sm: Local pain; disability
sg: Swelling; tenderness
cm: Growth deformity
xr: Displacement of epiphysis unusual

EPIPHYSEAL PLATE SEPARATION
at: Epiphyseal Plate Injury, Type I
et: Shearing or avulsion force, usually in children ages 10-16
sm: Local pain; disability
sg: Swelling; tenderness
cm: Prognosis excellent
xr: Complete separation of epiphysis from metaphysis without bony
fracture

EPIPHYSIS FRACTURE-SEPARATION, 1ST DEGREE
at: Epiphyseal Plate Injury, Type II
et: Shearing or avulsion force, usually in children ages 10-16
sm: Local pain; disability
sg: Swelling; tenderness
cm: Prognosis excellent
xr: Line of separation extends along epiphyseal plate for variable distance and then out through a portion of metaphysis

EPIPHYSIS FRACTURE-SEPARATION, 2ND DEGREE
at: Epiphyseal Plate Injury, Type III
et: Intra-articular shearing force, usually in children ages 10-16
sm: Local pain; disability

sg: Swelling; tenderness; deformity
cm: Prognosis good
xr: Fracture line extends from joint surface to weak zone of epiphyseal plate and then along the plate to its periphery

EPIPHYSIS FRACTURE-SEPARATION, 3RD DEGREE

at: Epiphyseal Plate Injury, Type IV
et: Intra-articular shearing force, usually in children ages 10-16
sm: Local pain; disability
sg: Swelling; tenderness
cm: Malunion; growth deformity
xr: Fracture line extends from joint surface through the epiphysis, across the full thickness of the epiphyseal plate, and through a portion of the metaphysis producing a complete split

EXTENSOR DIGITORUS LONGUS TENOSYNOVITIS (TOE)

et: Unknown; excessive forcible use of toe extensors as in running early in season; tight fitting shoes
sm: Pain over dorsum of foot and toes, especially on movement
sg: Tenderness, swelling, and crepitus over dorsum of foot and toes; pain elicited by active extension and passive flexion of toes and active dorsiflexion and passive plantarflexion of ankle
cm: Persistent disability; recurrence

EXTENSOR HALLUCIS LONGUS TENOSYNOVITIS

et: Unknown; possibly due to excessive forcible use of great toe extensor as in running early in season; tight fitting shoes
sm: Pain over foot and great toe, especially on movement
sg: Tenderness over dorsum of great toe; pain elicited by active extension and passive flexion of great toe and active dorsiflexion and passive plantarflexion of ankle
cm: Persistent disability; recurrence

EYE, CONJUNCTIVITIS, TRAUMATIC

et: Direct blow; foreign body abrasion; may be associated with wearing of contact lens
sm: Pain; photophobia
sg: Red, swollen conjunctivae
cm: Infection

EYE, CORNEAL INJURY

et: Trauma; thermal or chemical burn; foreign body abrasion; laceration; may be associated with wearing of contact lens
sm: Pain; lacrimation; impaired vision
sg: Evidence of trauma best visualized by dye
cm: Infection; ulcer; astigmatism

EYE, CORNEAL OPACITY

et: Trauma; infection; may be associated with wearing of contact lens
sm: Depression of visual acuity varying with size and location of opacity
sg: Opacity seen under slit-lamp

33

EYE, CORNEAL ULCER

et: Imbedded foreign body; trauma; may be associated with wearing of contact lens
sm: Pain; photophobia; lacrimation
sg: Blepharospasm; localized area of erosion
cm: Infection, suppuration; iritis; cyclitis; purulent iridocyclitis; loss of eye

EYE, GLOBE INJURY

at: Eyeball Injury
et: Penetrating wound; nonpenetrating contusion
sm: Severe pain; sensation of hot liquid escaping from eye; impaired vision; photophobia
sg: Variable according to extent of injury; evidence of trauma; hyphema; escape of intraocular fluid; shallowness or absence of anterior chamber; tear and prolapse of iris; dislocation of lens; detached retina; optic nerve injury
cm: Infection; iridocyclitis; ophthalmitis; glaucoma; blindness

EYE, IRIS INJURY

et: Trauma
sm: Pain; impaired vision; photophobia
sg: Dilatation of pupil; paralysis of accommodation; tear in iris; hyphema
cm: Residual impaired vision

EYE, PERIORBITAL HEMATOMA

at: Black Eye; Mouse; Shiner
et: Direct blow to periorbital rim or surrounding structures resulting in subcutaneous hemorrhage
sm: Local pain; possibly impaired vision
sg: Tenderness, swelling, ecchymosis of eyelids
cm: Occasionally associated with subcutaneous emphysema in presence of orbit fractures; conjunctivitis in severely swollen eyes

EYE, RETINAL DETACHMENT

at: Detached Retina
et: Trauma; choroidal hemorrhage; neoplasm; myopic degeneration; chorioretinitis; other causes
sm: Pain, sensation of flashing lights with trauma; impaired vision; later, appearance of dark cloud in visual field
cm: Blindness; secondary glaucoma
lb: Ophthalmoscopy: flat detachment: cloudiness of retina; tortuosity, diminution of reflex to light in vessels. Steep detachment: collection of gray-green folds first in periphery; tortuous vessels; visible hole or rent

FABELLA FRACTURE

et: Direct blow; violent contraction of gastrocnemius muscle
sm: Pain on posterolateral aspect of knee, especially on contraction of gastrocnemius
sg: Tenderness over affected area
cm: Disability
xr: Fracture of fabella; check opposite knee to rule out bipartite fabella

FACE CONTUSION

et: Direct blow to face
sm: Variable pain
sg: Swelling; ecchymosis; tenderness
xr: Fracture ruled out

FAT EMBOLISM

et: Embolization involving fat globules subsequent to extensive crushing injury to soft tissues and long bones or, less commonly, to extensive surgery on bone or fatty tissue; coalescing of liquid fat from ruptured fat cells to form globules in blood stream; small pulmonary capillaries plugged, resulting in acute obstruction of pulmonary circulation; some fat emboli bypass or pass through pulmonary bed to enter systemic circulation with widespread effect, especially in brain, skin, and kidneys
sm: Variable severity; If acute: sudden dyspnea, tachypnea beginning one or two days after injury. If not acute: restlessness, anxiety, progressing to delirium and coma; or, alternating periods of disorientation and lucidity for several days
sg: Obvious respiratory distress; cyanosis; petechiae on upper trunk, conjunctivae and retina visible after second or third day
cm: Death
lb: Fat globules in urine and sputum; elevated serum lipase
xr: Scattered small light densities throughout both lung fields

FAT PAD, INFRAPATELLAR, CONTUSION

at: Fat Pad Pinch
et: Direct trauma or impingement of pad; usually associated with other knee joint derangements
sm: Sharp twinge of pain with pendulum extension and on complete flexion of knee; history of discomfort
sg: Tenderness at patellar ligament just below inferior pole of patella; passive extension of knee is pain-free; knee instability upon weight bearing; mild effusion
cm: Traumatic arthritis; calcification; ossification; fibrosis
xr: May reveal complication; radio-opaque arthrography reveals encroachment of radiolucent area on intercondylar space

FELON

at: Finger Cellulitis; Whitlow
et: Infection of finger tip, usually staphylococcal; puncture by splinters, contaminated needles; may follow infected hematoma or contusion
sm: Throbbing pain
sg: Slight swelling, redness of pulpy tip of finger; wound may not be visible
cm: Osteomyelitis

FEMUR FRACTURE, GREATER TROCHANTER

et: Fall onto trochanter; violent abducting muscular action; kick from horse
sm: Pain localized in trochanteric region upon shifting of body weight; disability
sg: Tenderness and swelling localized in trochanteric region; loose fragment may be palpated; pain elicited by rotation and active ab-

duction of leg
cm: Persistent weakness in abduction of leg
xr: Separated fragment of greater trochanter of varying size; in adolescents, separation usually occurs at epiphyseal line and entire trochanter is displaced

FEMUR FRACTURE, HEAD

et: Direct blow as from fall
sm: Pain; stiffness; locking of hip; disability
sg: Bony crepitus on passive motion; local tenderness
cm: Traumatic arthritis; segmental aseptic necrosis of femoral head
xr: Linear crack of femoral head extending down into neck; or, detachment of marginal fragment

FEMUR FRACTURE, INTERCONDYLAR

at: "T" Fracture of Femur; Dicondylar Fracture of Femur
et: Direct blow as from fall onto foot or knee
sm: Local pain; disability
sg: Hemarthrosis, excess fluid in knee joint; marked swelling in lower half of thigh; variable amount of visible deformity and shortening of extremity; tenderness in supracondylar region extending around femur; fragment may be palpable beneath quadriceps tendon and in popliteal space; marked broadening of lower end of femur visible and palpable; condyles can be sqeezed together
cm: Severe and permanent disability if reduction not successful; chronic synovitis; injury to popliteal vessels and nerves
xr: Fracture through shaft plus vertical split in lower end of femur which ends below in intercondylar fossa; separation of condyles; articular portion rarely involved; distal end of proximal fragment may rest between the condyles so that one is tipped backward more than the other

FEMUR FRACTURE, LATERAL CONDYLE

et: Direct blow to lateral side of knee; fall from height onto feet; forcible adduction torsion action
sm: Pain; history of severe trauma; disability
sg: Hemarthrosis; swelling; no shortening; false motion toward side of lesion if due to pushing up of condyle, or away from side of lesion if due to avulsed lateral collateral ligament; localized tenderness; rarely possible to palpate fragments or contour abnormalities; possibly locking knee action
cm: Traumatic arthritis
lb: Aspiration shows fat particles in blood
xr: Fracture line vertical or roughly transverse, breaking lower end of condyle off; or condyle may be split in frontal plane thus separating its prominent posterior portion (rare); or, condyle may be shattered; or, small portion of lateral surface of condyle avulsed; displacement not marked, but may be slipped upward or downward or moderately rotated

FEMUR FRACTURE, LATERAL CONDYLE, CHONDRAL

et: Torsion injury with foot relatively internally rotated on femur; forcible relocation of dislocated or subluxated patella causing contusion of articular cartilage, fissuring, and complete chondral fracture

sm: Persistent pain; locking of knee; disability
sg: Swelling; hemarthrosis; crepitus; tenderness over lateral femoral condyle; possible abnormal patellar mobility
cm: Traumatic arthritis; residual joint dysfunction
xr: Ordinary films negative except "skyline" view may show abnormal patellofemoral relationship; radio-opaque arthrography may show radiolucent filling defect in knee joint

FEMUR FRACTURE, LATERAL CONDYLE, OSTEOCHONDRAL

et: Torsion injury with foot relatively internally rotated on femur; violent relocation of dislocated or subluxated patella, causing complete osteochondral fracture which may be pedunculated
sm: Locking of knee; persistent pain, disability
sg: Swelling; hemarthrosis; crepitus; tenderness over lateral femoral condyle; possible abnormal patellar mobility
cm: Traumatic arthritis; residual joint dysfunction
lb: Aspiration shows fat particles in blood
xr: Osteochondral fragment in knee joint; oblique films helpful if defect present on lateral aspect of condyle; "skyline" view may show abnormal patellofemoral relationship

FEMUR FRACTURE, LESSER TROCHANTER

et: Excessive forcible hyperextension and abduction of hip; sudden violent strain on iliopsoas muscle
sm: Pain in upper and inner aspects of thigh; disability
sg: Weakness of iliopsoas muscle; tenderness and swelling in upper and inner aspects of thigh; inability to flex hip actively in sitting position; pain elicited on hyperextension of hip
cm: Prolonged disability
xr: Entire lesser trochanteric avulsed upward from attachment to femur; in adolescents, epiphysis of lesser trochanter separated; views should be in moderate external rotation

FEMUR FRACTURE, MEDIAL CONDYLE

et: Direct blow on medial side of knee; fall from height onto feet; forcible abduction torsion of leg
sm: History of severe trauma; local pain; disability
sg: Hemarthrosis; swelling; no shortening; false motion only toward side of lesion if due to pushing up of condyle, or away from side of lesion if medial collateral ligament avulsed; local tenderness; knee may be locked
cm: Traumatic arthritis
lb: Aspiration shows fat particles in blood
xr: Fracture line vertical or roughly transverse, breaking lower end of condyle off; or, condyle may be split in frontal plane, separating its prominent posterior portion (rare); or, condyle may be shattered; or, small portion of medial surface of condyle avulsed; displacement not marked but may be slipped upward or downward or moderately rotated

FEMUR FRACTURE, MEDIAL CONDYLE, CHONDRAL

et: Torsion injury with foot externally rotated on femur; violent relocation of subluxated or dislocated patella, causing contusion of articular cartilage, fissuring, and complete chondral fracture

sm: Locking of knee; persistent pain, disability
sg: Swelling; hemarthrosis; crepitus; tenderness over medial femoral condyle
cm: Traumatic arthritis; residual joint dysfunction
xr: Ordinary films negative; radio-opaque arthrography may show radiolucent filling defect in knee joint

FEMUR FRACTURE, MEDIAL CONDYLE, OSTEOCHONDRAL

et: Torsion injury with foot externally rotated on femur; violent relocation of dislocated or subluxated patella, causing complete osteochondral fracture which may be pedunculated
sm: Locking of knee; persistent pain; disability
sg: Swelling; hemarthrosis; crepitus; tenderness
cm: Traumatic arthritis; residual joint dysfunction
lb: Aspiration shows fat particles in blood
xr: Osteochondral fragment in knee joint; corresponding defect in medial femoral condyle; oblique films helpful

FEMUR FRACTURE, NECK

at: Includes: Intracapsular Femur Fracture; Subcapital Femur Fracture; Transcervical Femur Fracture
et: Direct blow; fall from height
sm: Pain over front of hip upon leg motion; disability; inability to bear weight
sg: Leg in position of external rotation; shortening of extremity; swelling; ecchymosis; trochanter elevated
cm: Nonunion; aseptic necrosis of femoral head; shock
xr: May be impacted; fracture line runs transversely or slightly obliquely across neck at its middle narrowest portion or nearer the head; fracture line may be horizontal, oblique, or vertical; lower fragment pulled upward, outward and backward; head remains in acetabulum

FEMUR FRACTURE, POSTERIOR CONDYLE

et: Fall from height
sm: Pain over posterior aspect of knee upon movement; limited motion of knee; disability
sg: Tenderness localized to posterior aspect of knee; swelling
cm: Persistent disability, stiffness of knee; traumatic arthritis; avascular necrosis of fractured fragment
xr: Fracture consists of approximately posterior half inch of femoral condyle, usually the medial; displacement minimal

FEMUR FRACTURE, SHAFT

et: Direct blow; fall from height
sm: Pain; disability
sg: Shortening of extremity; tenderness; angular deformity; false motion; swelling; crepitus
cm: Severe shock; delayed union; malunion; nonunion; damage to femoral or popliteal vessels, sciatic or peroneal nerves; fat emboli
xr: Fracture may be roughly transverse, short or long oblique, spiral, comminuted, segmentally displaced, overriding, or rotated

FEMUR FRACTURE, SHAFT, FATIGUE

at: Femur March Fracture; Femur Stress Fracture
et: Forcible repetitive activity as in distance running, bowling; chronic adductor muscle strain
sm: Insidious onset of pain in inner aspect of mid-thigh; disability
sg: Vague tenderness at inner aspect of thigh; may be referred to groin or knee
xr: Incomplete fracture of medial aspect of femur at junction of upper and middle thirds; periosteal reaction

FEMUR FRACTURE, SUPRACONDYLAR

et: Direct blow; forcible torsion action; fall from height onto foot or knee
sm: Pain; history of severe injury followed by complete disability
sg: Hemarthrosis; excess fluid in knee joint; marked swelling in lower half of thigh; variable amount of visible deformity and shortening of extremity; tenderness in supracondylar region extending around femur; fragments may be palpated beneath quadriceps tendon and in popliteal space; patella may not be felt
cm: Chronic synovitis, stiffness of knee; injury to popliteal vessels and nerves
xr: Fracture line across shaft tends to be roughly transverse or slightly oblique from before backward; may be long oblique and extensively comminuted; short distal fragment tipped backward projecting into popliteal space; upward displacement with overriding of fragments; or lateral displacement of distal fragment

FEMUR FRACTURE, TROCHANTERIC

at: Includes: Extracapsular Femur Fracture; Intertrochanteric Femur Fracture; Transtrochanteric Femur Fracture; Basilar Neck Femur Fracture; Subtrochanteric Femur Fracture; Peritrochanteric Femur Fracture
et: Direct blow; fall from height
sm: Pain in hip on movement of extremity; disability; inability to bear weight
sg: Swelling; shortening of extremity; leg fixed in position of external rotation; trochanter elevated; tenderness; false motion; crepitus
cm: Nonunion; malunion; coxa vara deformity; shock
xr: Neck bent downward on shaft in varus position; fracture line begins in region of greater trochanter and passes inward and downward roughly parallel to intertrochanteric line to region of lesser trochanter; comminuted; lesser trochanter may be detached; femoral shaft may be split; proximal fragment abducted, flexed, and rotated outward; distal fragment drops backward and rotates outward

FEMUR FRACTURE-SEPARATION, DISTAL EPIPHYSIS

at: Femoral Lower Epiphysis Separation
et: Excessive forcible hyperextension and torsion injuries at knee; occurs between ages 10 and 16
sm: Pain around knee; disability
sg: Marked swelling of knee; may be obvious deformity; usually about one inch shortening; lower end of diaphysis may be palpable beneath skin in popliteal space; may palpate femur anterior to adductor tubercle on lower end of diaphysis; abnormal mobility of knee joint in all directions
cm: Damage to popliteal vessels and nerves; may be confused with sprain of medial collateral ligaments; growth deformity

39

xr: Distal femoral epiphysis displaced forward and upward and rests on lower end of shaft between it and patella; separation may be incomplete and epiphysis only partly displaced; stress films will show displacement of epiphysis rather than opening of joint medially

FEMUR FRACTURE-SEPARATION, PROXIMAL EPIPHYSIS

et: Trauma; forcible torsion action; direct blow; stepping into hole when running; attempting to save self from falling after tripping; endocrine disturbance predisposing; usually occurs in obese adolescent of Froelich type

sm: Sudden pain in hip, knee, or along inner side of thigh followed by complete inability to bear weight actively

sg: Swelling in Scarpa's triangle; slight shortening; thigh fixed in position of external rotation and slight adduction; active movements of hip impossible; passive movements may elicit soft cartilaginous crepitus

cm: Chronic pain; traumatic arthritis; disability

xr: Femoral head remains in acetabulum but femoral neck displaced upward and externally rotated; epiphyseal surface of head applied closely to posterior portion of end of neck.

FEMUR OSTEOCHONDRITIS DISSECANS, LATERAL CONDYLE

et: Trauma; impingement of adjacent surfaces; underlying constitutional disorders

sm: Vague pain in knee joint accentuated by activity and relieved by rest; recurrent episodes of effusion, instability, and locking

sg: Loose bodies may be palpated; synovial thickening; effusion; quadriceps atrophy; crepitus in patellofemoral joint during flexion and extension; subpatellar tenderness upon compression; firm pressure over lateral femoral condyle elicits exquisite tenderness; incongruity in articular surface of lateral femoral condyle may be palpated

cm: Persistent disability; traumatic arthritis

xr: Large crescentic cavity in lateral femoral condyle with separating fragment in situ best seen on tangential posteroanterior projection with knee semiflexed; later, loose body may be seen elsewhere in joint

FEMUR OSTEOCHONDRITIS DISSECANS, MEDIAL CONDYLE

et: Trauma; partial intra-articular fracture or subchondral fracture; impingement of adjacent surfaces caused by flexion and external rotation of tibia on femur; impingement action of prominent medial tubercle of tibial spine; underlying constitutional disorder

sm: Vague pain in joint accentuated by activity and relieved by rest; varying degrees of recurrent episodes of effusion, instability, and locking

sg: Synovial thickening with effusion; quadriceps atrophy; crepitus in patellofemoral joint during flexion and extension; subpatellar tenderness upon compression; pressure over medial femoral condyle elicits exquisite tenderness; incongruity in articular surface of medial femoral condyle may be palpated; loose bodies may be palpated at joint margin or in suprapatellar pouch

cm: Persistent disability; traumatic arthritis

xr: Large crescentic cavity in lateral aspect of medial femoral condyle

with separating fragment in situ best seen on tangential posteroanterior projection with knee semiflexed; later, loose body may be
seen elsewhere in joint

FEMUR, SLIPPING PROXIMAL EPIPHYSIS

at: Adolescent Coxa Vara
et: Trauma; vascular disturbances at epiphyseal line, endocrine deficiency and imbalance, perhaps faulty nutrition are predisposing
factors; disturbance of cartilage matrix or epiphyseal plate and/or
of adjacent bone formation; usually limited to 10-16 years of age
following rapid growth
sm: Progressive; fatigue after weight bearing; pain, stiffness, and limp;
eventually pain localized to anterior aspect of hip when limits of
range of motion are reached
sg: Progressive; shortening of extremity; internal rotation and abduction becomes restricted; if displacement marked, leg may assume
position of flexion, abduction, and external rotation; tenderness
about anterior and lateral aspects of hip
cm: Aseptic necrosis of femoral head; traumatic arthritis; permanent
disability
xr: Head of femur displaced on neck downward and backward; neck
retains its normal angle but may show posterior torsion; in pre-
slipped stage, epiphyseal line is abnormally wide and irregular;
after slipping, seen best on lateral view, displacement of neck upward and forward on head of femur so that lowest point of proximal end of neck projects as a beaklike process; upper part of neck
is lengthened, lower part is shortened, whole neck becomes bowed;
in quiescent stage, new bone may form between lower border of
neck and overhanging head; in residual stage, femoral head appears
quite atrophic, especially in its lower half, and neck is very thick
and short

FIBULA FRACTURE, HEAD

et: Direct blow; excessive forcible varus strain on knee
sm: Pain localized over fibular head; disability
sg: Tenderness and swelling about fibular head; may show adduction
stress instability
cm: Involvement of peroneal nerve, biceps femoris tendon, or lateral
collateral ligament
xr: Comminuted fracture of fibular head without gross displacement

FIBULA FRACTURE, NECK

et: Direct blow; excessive forcible torsion action
sm: Pain localized to lateral aspect of leg just below knee; disability
sg: Tenderness and swelling localized over lateral aspect of leg just
below knee; muscle spasm; crepitus on palpation of upper fibula
cm: Peroneal nerve injury
xr: Spiral, short oblique or transverse fracture

FIBULA FRACTURE, SHAFT

et: Direct blow to lateral side of leg; indirect forcible leverage action
sm: Pain on weight bearing; disability
sg: No shortening; tenderness localized over site of fracture; false
motion; crepitus usually not demonstrable; pain elicited by pressing
tibia and fibula together or by rotating ankle while knee is flexed

41

cm: Crossunion; usually associated with other injuries
xr: Transverse fracture

FIBULA FRACTURE, SHAFT, FATIGUE

at: Fibula Stress Fracture; Fibula March Fracture
et: Excessive repetitive pounding as from running on hard surface
sm: Pain and distress on function; usually localized above ankle or near neck of fibula; no history of injury; complaints persist and remain localized; disability
sg: Local tenderness; edema; occasional erythema
cm: Recurrence at other sites
xr: Early films negative; after about two weeks, transverse crack revealed across fibula at a point above ankle joint or below neck of fibula; possibly, callus formation with no fracture line may be seen; 6-8 weeks later, healed fracture and callus remodelling visible

FIBULA FRACTURE, UPPER END

at: Fibula Fracture, Proximal End
et: Direct blow
sm: Pain over upper fibular region upon weight bearing; disability
sg: Swelling and tenderness over upper fibular region; pain elicited by weight bearing, squeezing tibia and fibula together at middle of leg, rotating foot while knee is flexed, flexing leg against resistance
xr: Oblique or transverse fracture of upper fibula; little tendency to displacement of fragments; proximal fragment may be displaced upward and backward by pull of biceps tendon

FIBULA FRACTURE-DISLOCATION, UPPER END

et: Direct blow; forcible torsion action
sm: Pain localized over lateral aspect of leg at head of fibula; disability
sg: Tenderness and swelling localized over fibular head; deformity palpable; instability of fibular head
cm: Movability of fibular head by passive motion; involvement of peroneal nerve
xr: Fracture-dislocation of upper end of fibula

FIBULAR COLLATERAL LIGAMENT BURSITIS

at: Fibular Head Bursitis
et: Excessive forcible repetitive activity as in running
sm: Pain proximal to head of fibula, especially on extension of knee but not in active flexion against resistance
sg: Tenderness and diffuse swelling above head of fibula; palpation of fluctuant mass around head of fibula (rare)
cm: Peroneal nerve palsy; calcification; prone to recurrence; infection
pa: Inflammation of bursa between fibular collateral ligament and biceps femoris just adjacent to their fibular attachments

FINGER DISLOCATION, INTERPHALANGEAL

et: Forcible hyperextension; direct blow to interphalangeal capsule and ligaments
sm: Pain; disability
sg: Deformity; swelling; limitation of motion; instability
cm: Chronic instability; limited motion
xr: Chip fracture ruled out; dislocation demonstrated

FINGER FRACTURE, DISTAL PHALANX
et: Direct violence; crushing blow
sm: Throbbing pain
sg: Swelling, tenderness, cyanosis of finger tip
cm: Bone necrosis due to pressure; nonunion; rotary or angular deformity
xr: Comminution of distal phalanx

FINGER FRACTURE, MIDDLE PHALANX
et: Direct blow; indirect force
sm: Pain; disability
sg: Deformity; swelling; stiffness; crepitus
cm: Permanent deformity, stiffness
xr: If in distal portion, proximal fragment angulated volarward; if in proximal portion, proximal fragment pulled dorsalward by extensor retinaculum, distal fragment displaced forward with sublimus tendon

FINGER FRACTURE, PROXIMAL PHALANX
et: Direct blow, as in being stepped upon by cleats; may be from hyperextension, hyperflexion, or torsion forces
sm: Pain; disability
sg: Tenderness; swelling; crepitus
cm: Malunion of oblique-type fracture
xr: If central portion: fragment usually angulated volarward (hyperextension type); if distal portion: dorsal angulation with transverse fracture (hyperflexion type)

FINGER FRACTURE, "T" TYPE
et: Direct blow
sm: Pain; disability
sg: Tenderness; swelling; crepitus; stiffness
cm: Traumatic arthritis; anklyosis; angulation
xr: Intercondylar fracture of distal end of proximal or middle phalanx

FINGER SPRAIN, PROXIMAL INTERPHALANGEAL
at: Jammed Finger; Stoved Finger
et: Telescoping blow to finger
sm: Pain; disability
sg: Local tenderness, swelling; weakness; variable degree of severity of joint instability
cm: Permanent deformity, stiffness
.pa: Variable severity of injury to ulnar collateral ligament, less frequently to radial ligament

FLATFEET, SYMPTOMATIC
at: Fallen Arches; Weakfoot; Relaxed Foot
et: Congenital; ill-fitted shoes; muscle atrophy and loss of support; may follow rapid growth when muscle strength lags behind bony growth; obesity, excessive exercise adds stress
sm: Pain present in arch, frequently extending behind medial malleolus and radiating up leg to lower back; loss of spring in step; stiffness; disability
sg: Persistence of attitude of eversion during periods of weight-bearing; peroneal muscle spasm

cm: Calluses under medial side of heel; first metatarsophalangeal joint, and beneath prominent scaphoid bone

pa: Ligaments of longitudinal arch become weakened and relaxed; bony architecture changes

FLEXOR DIGITORUM LONGUS TENOSYNOVITIS (TOE)

et: Unknown; probably due to excessive forcible use of toe flexors as in running early in season

sm: Pain localized over plantar aspect of foot and behind medial malleolus; disability

sg: Pain elicited on active flexion and passive hyperextension of toes and active plantarflexion and passive dorsiflexion of ankle

cm: Persistent disability; recurrence

FLEXOR HALLUCIS LONGUS TENOSYNOVITIS

et: Unknown; probably due to excessive forcible use of great toe flexor as in running early in season

sm: Pain localized over plantar aspect of foot and deep behind ankle and anterior to achilles tendon; disability

sg: Pain elicited on active flexion and passive hyperextension of great toe and active plantarflexion and passive dorsiflexion of ankle

cm: Persistent disability; recurrence

FOOD POISONING, STAPHYLOCOCCAL

et: Ingestion of food containing staphylococcal enterotoxin: e.g., poorly refrigerated cream pastries, custards, cottage cheese, potato salad

sm: Onset 1-6 hours following meal; nausea; vomiting; abdominal cramps; diarrhea; sweating; headache; prostration; duration of acute symptoms 5-6 hours

sg: Shock; blood, mucus in stools; absence of fever

cm: Dehydration with acidosis

lb: Positive culture of feces, food

FOOT CONTUSION, PLANTAR

at: Bone Bruise; Stone Bruise

et: Direct trauma to plantar aspect of heel or ball of foot as by repeated pounding on hard surface, stepping on hard small object, faultily-placed spike, loose cleat, wrinkle in sock

sm: Persistent pain localized at site of trauma; varying disability

sg: Local tenderness; palpable nodule at site of trauma; boggy softening of subcutaneous tissues

cm: Circulatory, nerve, and lymph involvement possible as well as periosteal changes; calcification; prone to recurrence

FROSTBITE

et: Freezing of tissues from excessive exposure to cold; high winds, dampness, generalized chilling common contributing factors

sm: Progressive numbness, anesthesia; pricking sensation; mild to severe pain

sg: Yellowish white area of hard skin: subsequently, according to degree, erythema, livid cyanosis, blisters, pallor; sloughing of skin

cm: Gangrene; lowered local resistance to cold

pa: Hyperemia, edema, blistering, secondary thrombosis of small vessels, necrosis of skin and subcutaneous tissues

44

FURUNCULOSIS

at: Boils; Furuncles
et: Staphylococcal infection of hair follicles, sebaceous glands; areas of friction common sites of involvement; poor hygiene contributory; diabetes mellitus predisposing; communicable via direct contact or indirect contamination
sm: Local pain; malaise; stiffness
sg: Tender, erythematous, nodular swelling with hair follicle in center; fluctuation, suppuration, central necrotic core; fever
cm: Carbuncle; lymphangitis; lymphadenitis; septicemia

GALEAZZI'S FRACTURE

at: Piedmont Fracture
et: Fall onto outstretched hand
sm: Local pain, disability
sg: Deformity; swelling; tenderness; crepitus on motion over distal radioulnar area
cm: Malunion; nonunion
xr: Fracture of distal radius with dorsal subluxation of ulna at distal radioulnar joint

GANGLION

at: Synovial Hernia; Synovial Cyst
et: Trauma; degenerative changes
sm: Pain; frequently asymptomatic; mild disability
sg: Possible tenderness over site; palpable cystic mass, usually on wrist or dorsum of foot
pa: Defect in fibrous sheath of a joint with synovial outpouching

GASTROENTERITIS, ACUTE

et: Infection; usually virus, escherichia coli, salmonella, or shigella
sm: Onset sudden; abdominal pain; vomiting; sometimes preceded by malaise, anorexia, nausea; diarrhea
sg: Mild type: moderate fever for 1-2 days; dehydration. Febrile type: high fever, prostration
lb: Pus in stools; positive culture from stools

GINGIVITIS

et: Infection; malocclusion; impacted food, calculus; poor oral hygiene; poorly fitted prosthesis or protective mouth guard
sm: Usually asymptomatic; sometimes slight bleeding on minor trauma
sg: Bright red, inflamed gum; evidence of bleeding
cm: Periodontitis
pa: Inflammation of gum tissue

GLENOHUMERAL DISLOCATION, ANTERIOR

at: Subcoracoid Dislocation
et: Leverage force on abducted arm, as in making an arm tackle; less frequently, a fall or blow to shoulder from rear
sm: Pain; disability
sg: Arm fixed in slight abduction and external rotation; axilla broadened with anterior axillary fold displaced downward; deformity with acromion prominent and deltoid flattened; head of humerus palpable in abnormal position

cm: Associated fractures of humerus, scapula; nerve, vascular injury
xr: Head of humerus in subcoracoid position, no longer in contact with glenoid fossa; fracture ruled out

GLENOHUMERAL DISLOCATION, DOWNWARD

at: Subglenoid Dislocation
et: Leverage force on abducted arm, as in making an arm tackle
sm: Pain; disability
sg: Deformity with deltoid flattened and head of humerus displaced downward; head of humerus palpated in axilla; arm fixed at about 45° abduction
cm: Associated fractures of humerus, scapula; nerve, vascular injury
xr: Downward dislocation demonstrated; fracture ruled out

GLENOHUMERAL DISLOCATION, POSTERIOR

at: Posterior Shoulder Dislocation
et: Leverage force applied to adducted arm as in fall forward onto hand; direct trauma to front of shoulder (rare)
sm: Pain; disability
sg: Arm fixed in adduction and internal rotation; swelling, especially posteriorly; deformity with acromion prominent and anterior deltoid flattened; diagnosis may be difficult
xr: Axillary view essential to show posteriorly displaced humerus head; fracture ruled out

GLENOHUMERAL SUBLUXATION, ANTERIOR, RECURRENT

at: Anterior Recurrent Shoulder Subluxation
et: Leverage force on abducted arm, as in making an arm tackle; forced abduction and external rotation as in throwing, backstroke
sm: Pain; momentary disability, sensation of shoulder slipping out of place; usually spontaneous relief with change of position of arm
sg: Before reduction, obvious deformity with humerus head prominent anteriorly; marked muscle spasm; loss of function. After reduction, sense of uneasiness on forced abduction and external rotation of arm; head of humerus palpable slipping against glenoid rim
cm: Dislocation; chronic instability

GLENOHUMERAL SUBLUXATION, POSTERIOR, RECURRENT

at: Recurrent Posterior Shoulder Subluxation
et: Flexion of shoulder to 50-60° in presence of lax posterior capsule
sm: Momentary pain, disability; thumping sensation on forward flexion of shoulder localized to posteroinferior aspect; usually spontaneous relief with change of arm position
sg: Before reduction, humerus head may be prominent posteriorly; slight flattening of anterior deltoid; muscle spasm; loss of function. After reduction, uneasiness on forced flexion
cm: Dislocation; chronic instability

GLUTEUS MEDIUS STRAIN

et: Excessive forcible abduction of hip as in gymnastics
sm: Pain in greater trochanteric region radiating proximally toward iliac crest; disability

sg: Grade by degree of severity: local tenderness and swelling; pain elicited on active hip abduction against resistance
cm: Chronicity

GRACILIS STRAIN

et: Excessive forcible flexion of hip as in doing splits
sm: Pain along edge of pubic ramus radiating along inner aspect of thigh; disability
sg: Grade by degree of severity: local tenderness and swelling; pain elicited on passive abduction of thigh; ecchymosis; defect may be palpable
cm: Persistent disability; prone to recurrence
xr: May show small downward avulsed fragment of bone from pubic ramus

GRANULOMA, SWIMMING POOL

et: Unknown; Mycobacterium balnei; presence of silica in water; granuloma development at site of healed abrasion usually 5-6 weeks following injury
sg: Single or multiple skin lesions; soft papules with possible ulceration; usual sites: nose, knees, elbows; spontaneous healing in 3-9 months
cm: Reinfection
lb: Mycobacterium balnei rarely isolated; tissue sections; tuberculin tests become positive

GROIN CONTUSION

et: Direct blow to groin
sm: Variable; disability, especially on running
sg: Pain elicited by passive extension and abduction of hip
cm: Damage to femoral vessels, femoral nerve, inguinal canal, spermatic cord and iliospoas muscle

HAMSTRING STRAIN

at: Pulled Hamstring
et: Muscular discoordination: poor body mechanics, altering stride, inadequate warmup, fatigue cramps; sudden violent stretch or contraction
sm: Sudden acute pain, subsequent discomfort at area of involvement; disability
sg: Grade by degree of severity: tenderness to tenseness at area of involvement, usually at ischial tuberosity, middle of posterior aspect of thigh or popliteal region; gap or bunching may be palpable; possibly hematoma
cm: Prolonged disability; recurrence
xr: May show avulsion fracture at ischial tuberosity or head of fibula

HAMSTRING TENOSYNOVITIS

et: Excessive unaccustomed activity
sm: Pain behind knee; disability
sg: Tenderness, mild swelling; possible crepitus behind knee; pain elicited by active flexion of knee or on passive straight leg raising
cm: Persistent disability

HAY FEVER
at: Allergic Rhinitis; Pollenosis
et: Hypersensitive reaction to pollen and other antigens; seasonal recurrence; familial tendency
sm: Sneezing, rhinorrhea; intense pruritus of eyes, nose; lacrimation; frontal headache
sg: Nasal mucosa congestion; nasal discharge; conjunctivitis
cm: Asthma; secondary infection
lb: Nasal smear shows increased eosinophils; skin test identifies allergen

HEART, AORTA COARCTATION
et: Congenital
sm: May be asymptomatic if inactive; persistent headaches; numbness and weakness in legs
sg: Elevated blood pressure in upper extremities compared to lower; evidence of increased collateral circulation such as pulsations along ribs, interscapular area, and supraclavicular area
cm: Contraindication to activity; poor prognosis if untreated; cardiac decompensation and hypertension
xr: Notching of ribs; enlarged left ventricle
pa: Constriction of aorta at or below the entrance of the obliterated ductus arteriosus, usually just distal to the origin of the left subclavian artery

HEART, AORTIC VALVE STENOSIS, CONGENITAL
et: Congenital subaortic stenosis; congenital fusion or defect of aortic cusps
sm: May be asymptomatic; exertional dyspnea; orthopnea; dizziness; syncope; anginal pain
sg: Harsh systolic mumur in aortic area transmitted to neck with corresponding thrill; apical thrust; aortic second sound diminished or absent; low volume of pulse, rising slowly (plateau-pulse)
cm: Contraindication for exertional sport, having been associated with sudden death from participation; angina pectoris; congestive heart failure
lb: EKG: QRS usually normal; R wave high in left precordial leads; if severe, S-T segment depressed, T wave inverted. Catheterization of left side demonstrates increase in gradient of pressure across aortic valve in systole
xr: Dilatation of ascending aorta; enlargement of left atrium, left ventricle

HEART, AORTIC VALVE STENOSIS, RHEUMATIC
et: Rheumatic fever
sm: Syncope with exertion; angina pectoris
sg: Systolic murmur in 2nd interspace, transmitted into neck; 2nd aortic sound diminished or absent; cardiac reserve limited, fixed
cm: Congestive cardiac failure, refractory to treatment; contraindicated for exertional sports, having been associated with sudden death from participation

HEART, INTERVENTRICULAR SEPTAL DEFECTS
et: Congenital
sm: Variable; cyanosis; intolerance to exertion
sg: Loud blowing systolic murmur heard over the precordium; in-

creased 2nd pulmonic sound
pa: Defect of variable size in the interventricular septum near apex of heart

HEART, MITRAL VALVE INSUFFICIENCY

at: Mitral Valve Regurgitation
et: Congenital; rheumatic endocarditis; subacute bacterial endocarditis
sm: May be asymptomatic; dyspnea; cough; weakness, fatigability; palpitation
sg: Apical 1st sound often replaced by loud blowing holosystolic murmur extending into axilla, back, softer with inspiration; systolic thrill; apical beat strong, displaced downward to left; accentuation of 2nd pulmonic sound; 3rd cardiac sound frequently heard
cm: Congestive heart failure
lb: EKG demonstrates deviation of left axis; possible atrial fibrillation
xr: Enlargement of left atrium, ventricle; systolic expansion of left atrium; calcification of mitral valve

HEART, MITRAL VALVE STENOSIS

et: Rheumatic heart disease; congenital
sm: Dyspnea; cough; weakness; hemoptysis
sg: Apical beat displaced to left; systolic thrust left of sternum; pre-systolic or early diastolic rumble of crescendo type, medial to cardiac apex, elicited after exercise while lying on left side; rumble absent with atrial fibrillation; loud, staccato, high pitched, snapping 1st sound at apex; 2nd pulmonic sound exaggerated; duration of murmur suggests degree of stenosis; distention of cervical veins; later, pulmonary congestion; edema of ankles
cm: Congestive cardiac failure; atrial fibrillation; peripheral or pulmonary embolism; pulmonary infarction; bacterial endocarditis
lb: EKG: vertical axis of QRS; right deviation infrequent; P waves large, broad, notched, especially in Leads I, II; P waves broad, diphasic in Lead V_1

HEART, MYOCARDIAL INFARCTION

at: Coronary Thrombosis
et: Thrombosis secondary to coronary atherosclerosis; congenitally poor collateral circulation to myocardium
sm: Severe, crushing substernal pain; cold sweating; possibly nausea, vomiting; possibly dyspnea; anxiety
sg: Obvious distress; prostration; tachycardia; pulse possibly irregular; gallop rhythm; 4th cardiac sound; hypotension; shock; fever; rales
cm: Acute pulmonary edema; heart failure; pulmonary embolism caused by mural thrombus; cardiac aneurysm; rupture of heart; arrhythmias; recurrence
lb: EKG demonstrates anterior infarct revealing abnormal Q waves, elevation of RS-T segment, inversion of T wave in Leads I, AVL, left precordial leads; or, inferior infarct revealing similar changes in Leads II, III, AVF; increase in white blood cells; elevation of serum enzymes
pa: Myocardial necrosis

HEART, MYOCARDIUM CONTUSION

et: Direct blow to chest as in baseball, football, or boxing
sm: Local pain
sg: Tachycardia; fibrillation of auricles, ventricles; arrhythmia

49

cm: Cardiac failure; rupture of myocardium; myocardial infarction; aneurysm; valvular incompetence; perforation of septum; traumatic pericarditis, tamponade; death

lb: EKG: flattening or inversion of T waves; deviation of S-T segment; heart electrically unstable

HEART, PATENT DUCTUS ARTERIOSUS

et: Congenital anomaly connecting aorta and pulmonary artery

sm: May be asymptomatic; exertional dyspnea

sg: Continuous "machinery" murmur during both systole and diastole; loud 2nd pulmonary sound

cm: Cardiac failure; possibly subacute bacterial endocarditis

xr: Accentuated pulmonary conus; increased vascular lung markings

HEART, PERICARDITIS, ACUTE

et: Bacterial or viral infection; trauma

sm: Sharp or dull precordial pain radiating to left shoulder, neck, arm, or epigastrium; orthopnea; chills; weakness; anxiety

sg: Obvious distress; pallor or cyanosis; fever, possibly with delirium. If fibrinous: superficial, harsh pericardial friction-rub near left border of lower sternum. If serofibrinous: faint cardiac sounds; pericardial friction-rub limited to base of heart

cm: Cardiac tamponade; myocardial failure

lb: Polymorphonuclear leukocytosis; anemia; EKG: elevated S-T segment in Leads I, II; elevated R-T segment; T wave flattened at return of S-T to isoelectric line; inverted T wave in 3 leads; diminution of QRS voltage

xr: Outline of cardiac chambers usually well demarcated, normal; obliteration of greater vessels; enlargement of heart silhouette; vascular pedicle widened; indistinct segmentation along left contour; diminution or absence of pulsations

HEART, PULMONARY VALVE INSUFFICIENCY

et: Association with mitral stenosis, congenital heart disease, bacterial endocarditis, rheumatic cardiac disease (rare)

sm: Variable; exertional dyspnea; cough

sg: Blowing, early diastolic murmur in 2nd, 3rd interspaces; systolic murmur frequent in pulmonary area; accentuation of 2nd pulmonary sound; cyanosis

cm: Cardiac failure

lb: Catheterization demonstrates marked elevation of pressure in pulmonary artery; EKG demonstrates right ventricular strain

xr: Right ventricular hypertrophy; dilatation of pulmonary artery

HEART, PULMONARY VALVE STENOSIS

at: Pulmonic Stenosis

et: Congenital; possibly rheumatic fever, subacute bacterial endocarditis

sm: Possibly asymptomatic until early adult life; exertional dyspnea; fatigability

sg: Right ventricular heave; harsh systolic murmur over pulmonary area, combined with weak or absent pulmonic 2nd sound at base; thrill in pulmonic area and suprasternal notch; enlarged, pulsatile liver; engorged vessels in neck

cm: Congestive cardiac failure

lb: Hematocrit elevated; circulation time prolonged; oxygen saturation normal; EKG: deviation of right axis; strain of right ventricle; incomplete right bundle branch block; T waves broad, elevated

xr: Right ventricular hypertrophy; dilatation of pulmonary artery; pulmonary conus full; pulsation at hilus minimal

HEART, RHEUMATIC DISEASE, ACTIVE

at: Rheumatic Heart Disease, Active

et: Infection by Beta hemolytic streptococcus (group A) followed by rheumatic fever

sm: Precordial pain; palpitation; dyspnea; cough; weakness

sg: Obvious distress; fever; tachycardia; arrhythmia; systolic or diastolic murmur; pericardial friction-rub; gallop rhythm. Pericarditis: precordial friction-rub; dullness; bronchial breathing at left scapula

cm: Atrial fibrillation; adhesive pericarditis; congestive heart failure; recurrence

lb: EKG: prolonged P-R interval; partial atrioventricular block; bundle-branch block; QRS complex notched or slurred; transient alteration of T wave

xr: Enlarged heart

pa: Inflammation of endocardium, myocardium, and/or pericardium with possible fibrosis

HEART, TACHYCARDIA, ATRIAL PAROXYSMAL

et: Ectopic stimuli arising in atria; emotional stress; hyperthyroidism; severe infection; unknown

sm: Variable: sudden onset of pounding in chest, throat; lasts minutes to hours; nausea; dizziness; weakness; syncope

sg: Rapid, regular cardiac beat; may be terminated by Valsalva maneuver, pressure on eyeball, or carotid sinus; cyanosis; hypotension

cm: Cardiac neurosis; myocardial infarct; congestive failure in prolonged attacks

lb: Increased circulation-time; reduced cardiac output, vital capacity; EKG: series of premature atrial beats; abnormal P waves, normal QRS at 150-220 per minute; Wenckebach phenomenon possible; P-R interval usually lengthened

HEART, TACHYCARDIA, SINUS

et: Unknown; usually extracardiac causes such as emotional stress, exercise. Extreme tachycardia: elevation of body temperature; anemia; acute myocardial injury; thyrotoxicosis; conditions causing circulatory collapse; sympathomimetic drugs

sm: Possibly asymptomatic; dyspnea; palpitation; fatigue

sg: Rhythmic resting heart rate exceeding 100 per minute; little response to pressure on carotid sinus

lb: EKG demonstrates shortening of P-P intervals below 0.6 second; P waves recurring at regular intervals, each followed by QRS complex

HEAT EXHAUSTION

at: Heat Syncope; Heat Prostration

et: Unaccustomed exertion in hot, humid environment; dehydration; excessive loss of sodium through sweat; inability to dissipate generated body heat; deficient repletion of salt and water

sm: Fatigue; lassitude; faintness; palpitation; nausea; vomiting; headache; dyspnea; vertigo; dimness or blurring of vision; cramps; syncope

sg: State of shock; profuse sweating; rapid pulse; low blood pressure; ashen cold, wet skin; stupor

cm: Fatigue predisposing to traumatic injury in sports; possible progression into heat stroke

pa: Depletion of extracellular sodium chloride electrolytes

HEAT RASH

at: Prickly Heat Rash; Miliaria Rubra
et: Poral occlusion due to excessive sweating with minimal evaporation
sm: Pruritus
sg: Discrete, closely packed, red, pinhead-sized vesicopapules surrounded by red halo; each papule represents site of sweat pore
cm: Recurrence

HEAT STROKE

at: Sunstroke
et: Unaccustomed exertion in hot, humid environment; dehydration; inability to dissipate generated body heat; excessive body weight loss, obesity predisposing; eventually failure of temperature regulatory mechanism
sm: Sensation of extreme heat; mental confusion; headache; vertigo; photophobia; collapse
sg: Cessation of sweating; warm, dry skin; high fever increasing to above 105° if unchecked by emergency cooling measures; low blood pressure; rapid, weak, diminishing pulse; decrease of tendon reflexes; dilation of pupils; stertorous breathing; delirium; coma
cm: Death or irreversible brain damage from high fever; lessened tolerance to heat stress, possible, even with uneventful recovery

HEMATOCELE, TUNICA VAGINALIS, TRAUMATIC

et: Trauma
sm: Local pain
sg: Ecchymosis; doughy or solid swelling in cord or testicular area; not translucent
cm: Sterility

HEMORRHOIDS, THROMBOSED

at: Piles
et: Constipation; straining at stool; heavy lifting; sudden exertional effort; increased intra-abdominal pressure; idiopathic; familial tendency
sm: Pain, especially on defecation; pruritus
sg: External: lesion below pectinate line rounded, purplish; multiple thromboses; edema of anal tissue, ulceration, sloughing; bleeding with involvement of skin. Internal: rectal bleeding; protrusion following defecation; pain accentuated by palpation; later, prolapse of hemorrhoidal tissue; frequently resolved with no residual
lb: Anoscopy: mucosa indurated, ulcerated, discolored, prolapsed

HEPATITIS, INFECTIOUS

at: Epidemic Hepatitis; Yellow Jaundice
et: Virus; transmission through food, water contaminated usually from fecal matter; poor hygienic conditions

sm: Preicteric phase: asymptomatic; headache; malaise; anorexia; constipation; occasionally nausea, vomiting. Icteric phase: jaundice; pruritus; abdominal pain; tenderness in right upper quandrant; loss of weight
sg: Fever: hepatomegaly; splenomegaly; enlargement of posterior cervical lymphatic nodes
lb: Liver function tests abnormal; bile in urine; stools clay-colored

HERNIA, INGUINAL, DIRECT

et: Congenitally weak posterior inguinal wall; increased abdominal pressure precipitating hernia directly through wall; may first appear with exertion
sm: Usually painless inguinal swelling; reduction in recumbency; dragging sensation
sg: Visible, palpable mass protruding through posterior wall; less common than indirect hernia
cm: Recurrence; incarceration and intestinal obstruction (rare)

HERNIA, INGUINAL, INDIRECT

et: Failure of processus vaginalis to obliterate; resulting diverticulum at abdominal inguinal ring; physical exertion, increased abdominal pressure precipitating hernia along course of inguinal canal
sm: Painful inguinal lump relieved by recumbency; dragging sensation; may be asymptomatic
sg: Visible, palpable mass, may be scrotal; sac in inguinal canal demonstrated on cough
cm: Incarceration; strangulation; intestinal obstruction

HERNIA, MUSCLE

at: Fascial Hernia
et: Trauma; excessive physical activity; congenital defect
sm: Mild pain on activity; muscle easily fatigued
sg: Fusiform bulges appear in long axis of muscle on vigorous contraction, usually in lower extremity; defect variable in size; usually reducible
cm: Disability; secondary entrapment neuropathy
pa: Herniation of muscle tissue through defect in fascial sheath; or, muscle hypertrophy distends fascial compartment which then may become weak and split

HERNIA, UMBILICAL

at: Exomphalos
et: Congenital defect at umbilicus with superimposed increase in intra-abdominal pressure
sm: Pain; disorders of upper gastrointestinal tract
sg: Presence of mass at umbilicus; usually reducible
cm: Intestinal obstruction; incarceration; strangulation

HERPES SIMPLEX

et: Virus; Primary stage: usually occurs in first five years of life; communicable by direct transmission through break in skin or mucous membrane. Recurrent attacks: virus lying latent in tissues activated by sunburn, skin abrasion, emotional disturbance, fatigue, infection, or other precipitating agents

sm: Primary: malaise. Recurrent: mild pain, cosmetic discomfort
sg: Superficial vesicles on erythematous base, affecting skin or mucosa, usually on lip ("cold sore"); vesicles rupture, forming crusts; self-limited course
cm: Secondary infection; keratoconjunctivitis; visceral disease; encephalitis (rare)
lb: Leukocyte count normal; isolation of virus; eosinophilic intranuclear inclusions in tissue or fluid of vesicle; rising titer of specific neutralizing antibodies (primary)

HERPES SIMPLEX, TRAUMATIC

at: Herpes Simplex Gladiatorum
et: Virus communicable by direct transmission through minute abrasions of skin as in body-to-body contact in wrestling
sm: Variable but more severe than customary herpetic infections; malaise; chills; headache; sore throat; pain localized to lesions
sg: Maculopapular lesions turning into vesicles with crusts resembling impetigo; lesions clearing in 1-3 weeks; regional lymphadenopathy
cm: Secondary infection; keratoconjunctivitis; visceral lesions; encephalitis (rare); epidemic among wrestling squads
lb: Stained scrapings from vesicles

HIP DISLOCATION, ANTERIOR

et: Trauma; forcible abduction and external rotation of hip as from fall onto feet or knees; crushing injury to back or pelvis with hip in abduction
sm: Severe pain; disability
sg: Thigh maintained in position of abduction and external rotation, perhaps slight flexion or extension; head of femur palpable in abnormal position; lateral surface of hip flattened; greater trochanter displaced inward
cm: Conversion to posterior dislocation, associated fractures; rupture of femoral vessels; contusion of femoral or obturator nerve; aseptic necrosis of head of femur; traumatic arthritis
xr: Femoral head resting upon body of pubis, or on obturator foramen, or in perineal region or infracotyloid

HIP DISLOCATION, POSTERIOR

et: Violent force which approximates knee and pelvis causing flexed thigh into internal rotation and adduction; or, with hip flexed, strong backward thrust on femur may snap head out of acetabulum posteriorly
sm: Severe pain; inability to bear weight or move limb; disability
sg: Hip fixed in abnormal position of flexion, adduction, and internal rotation; apparent shortening of limb; trochanter unusually prominent; buttock on affected side unusually prominent; head of femur palpable in its abnormal position beneath glutei; tenderness on passive motion
cm: Shock; sciatic nerve palsy; traumatic arthritis; aseptic necrosis of femoral head
xr: Femoral head out of acetabulum resting high on posterior surface of ilium or low on ischium; lesser trochanter not visible; lateral or oblique views helpful

HIP OSTEOCHONDRITIS DISSECANS

et: Trauma; impingement of articular surfaces; underlying constitutional disorder sm: Not detached: aching after use, recurrent swelling. Detached: recurrent sudden locking accompanied by sharp pain and followed by effusion

sg: Crepitus, tenderness with passive motion; restriction of motion, especially internal rotation and abduction

cm: Traumatic arthritis; persistent disability

xr: Shallow excavation in articular surface of femoral head with discrete bone fragment lying either within the cavity or elsewhere in joint

pa: Segment of articular surface of femoral head deprived of blood supply; line of demarcation formed and avascular fragment separated

HIP POINTER

at: Iliac Crest Contusion

et: Direct blow at or above iliac crest; inadequate or illfitted hip pads contributory in football

sm: Pain, especially upon coughing; pain, tingling, burning in extremity on involved side; limitation of function

sg: Exquisite tenderness over iliac crest

xr: Avulsion fracture ruled out

HIP, SNAPPING

at: Clicking Hip

et: Unknown; chronic trochanteric bursitis with bursal thickening may be contributory

sm: Usually not painful but annoying and distressing, especially to hurdlers

sg: With knee flexed, active internal rotation of hip causes snapping noise

xr: Calcification of trochanteric bursa

pa: Slipping of fibrous band of deep surface of gluteus maximus over greater trochanter; or, tensor fasciae femoris sliding over trochanter

HIP SPRAIN

et: Excessive forcible torsion of extremity

sm: Pain in groin, occasionally in buttocks or lateral aspect of hip, intensified by motion or weight bearing

sg: Grade by degree of severity: flexion position assumed with body bent forward; decided limp; muscle spasm; decreased abduction and/or internal rotation of hip; tenderness and possibly swelling

cm: Persistent disability

HIP STRAIN

et: Excessive forcible repetitive use of hip external rotators

sm: Pain near posterior margin of greater trochanter radiating across buttocks to ischial tuberosity, especially on running or jumping; disability

sg: Grade by degree of severity: local tenderness; pain elicited by active external rotation or passive internal rotation of hip

cm: Chronicity

HIVES

at: Allergic Urticaria

et: Release of histamine from mast cell due to antigenic inhalants, injectants, foods, or external contactants sm: Variable; pruritus, pricking sensation during early formation of fluid in wheal; dyspnea; abdominal pain; hoarseness with mucosal involvement

sg: Transient erythematous or whitish swellings in skin; wheals; lesions, oval or round, enlarging by peripheral extension becoming confluent; rales with accentuated breath sounds

cm: Edema of larynx; anaphylactic shock

lb: Cutaneous testing in chronic cases of virtually no value

HUMERUS, EPICONDYLITIS, LATERAL

at: Radiohumeral Bursitis

et: Repeated sudden jerky, vigorous pronating movement of extended forearm and wrist, as in tennis strokes

sm: Pain in elbow, first intermittent, later persistent, radiating to forearm, wrist, possibly fingers; grip causes sharp pain

sg: Local tenderness over front of external epicondyle; pain with extension of hand against resistance; lack of pain with flexion against resistance

cm: Chronicity

xr: Occasional calcification in aponeurosis

pa: Strain of common extensor tendon; inflammation of aponeurosis, periosteum

HUMERUS EPICONDYLITIS, MEDIAL

et: Repeated sudden jerky, vigorous supinating movement of forearm and wrist as in throwing

sm: Pain on medial side of elbow, radiating to forearm, wrist, possibly fingers; weakness of hand; grip causes sharp pain

sg: Local tenderness; occasional swelling

xr: Occasional calcification adjacent to medial epicondyle

pa: Strain of common flexor tendon

HUMERUS FRACTURE, DICONDYLAR

at: Transverse Fracture, Distal Humerus

et: Direct violence to olecranon or posterior surface of ulna

sm: Elbow pain; disability

sg: Swelling; palpable deformity; false motion; crepitus

cm: Limitation of normal motion; ankylosis

xr: Fracture line lies just above epiphyseal line, coursing transversely through condyles; always partly intra-articular as it passes through coronoid and olecranon fossae

HUMERUS FRACTURE, GREATER TUBEROSITY

et: Direct violence; blow to shoulder; compression by acromion in hyperabduction injuries; forcible muscular avulsive action

sm: Pain, especially on internal rotation of shoulder; inability to abduct arm

sg: Acute tenderness and swelling over lateral surface of shoulder; crepitus on passive abduction or rotation

xr: Fracture demonstrated

HUMERUS FRACTURE, LATERAL EPICONDYLE

at: External Epicondyle Fracture

et: Direct violence; excessive forcible adduction of extended forearm

sm: Pain; limited motion

sg: Weakness in forearm supination and extension of wrist; swelling; localized tenderness
xr: Bony fragment displaced downward and forward

HUMERUS FRACTURE, MEDIAL EPICONDYLE

at: Internal epicondyle fracture; epitrochlear fracture; epiphyseal fracture of medial epicondyle
et: Forced abduction of extended elbow; direct violence
sm: Pain; limited motion
sg: Weakness in forearm pronation and flexion of wrist; swelling; joint tenderness
cm: Ulnar nerve injury
xr: Bony fragment displaced downward, forward, and rotated; avulsed fragment may be displaced into joint

HUMERUS FRACTURE, MEDIAL EPICONDYLAR EPIPHYSEAL AVULSION

at: Little League Elbow
et: Excessive repetitive vigorous stress on flexor-pronator muscles while throwing baseball, usually between ages 9-14
sm: Pain when flexing, pronating forearm
sg: Swelling; local tenderness
cm: Permanent limitation of movement
xr: Partial or complete avulsion of medial epicondylar epiphysis; loss of fascial markings suggesting edema, hematoma

HUMERUS FRACTURE, NECK, ABDUCTION

et: Force transmitted to upper end of humerus during arm abduction; occurs only with bony maturity
sm: Pain; limitation of motion; disability
sg: Deformity; swelling; ecchymosis; tenderness; crepitus
xr: Fracture line impacted at outer angle, open at inner angle

HUMERUS FRACTURE, NECK, ADDUCTION

et: Fall with arm at side with shearing force; occurs only with bony maturity
sm: Local pain; limitation of motion
sg: Swelling, ecchymosis; point tenderness; crepitus; may have abnormal mobility
xr: Fracture line open laterally, closed medially; inner cortex impacted into base of humeral head

HUMERUS FRACTURE, NECK EPIPHYSIS

at: Epiphyseal Separation, Proximal Humerus
et: Fall onto shoulder, elbow, or outstretched hand
sm: Local pain; limitation of motion
sg: Deformity; tenderness; shortening or distortion of anterior axillary fold; swelling
xr: Displacement of upper end of humeral shaft anterolaterally and superiorly

HUMERUS FRACTURE, SHAFT

et: Direct violence; fall onto arm at side; forcible muscular action as in throwing or hand wrestling
sm: Local pain; disability

57

sg: Shortening of humerus; swelling; abnormal mobility; crepitus
cm: Radial nerve injury; vascular injuries; nonunion; angular, rotary deformity
xr: Lower fragment usually drawn upward; if fracture is above deltoid insertion, lower fragment is drawn outward and upper fragment drawn inward

HUMERUS FRACTURE, SUPRACONDYLAR, EXTENSION
et: Fall onto hand with elbow flexed; less frequently, forced hyperextension of elbow
sm: Local pain; disability
sg: Local swelling; deformity; tenderness above condyles; false motion; crepitus
cm: Nerve, vascular injury; traumatic myositis ossificans; Volkmann's ischemic contracture
xr: Short distal fragment displaced upward and backward, may be rotated and displaced either medially or laterally

HUMERUS FRACTURE, SUPRACONDYLAR, FLEXION
et: Direct trauma to olecranon or posterior surface of ulna, usually by fall onto flexed elbow
sm: Local pain; disability
sg: Local swelling, tenderness; upper end of distal fragment may be palpable in front of elbow beneath biceps; cardinal bony points of elbow displaced anteriorly to line of humerus shaft; false motion; crepitus
xr: Proximal portion of distal fragment is displaced forward, may be rotated and displaced either medially or laterally

HYDROCELE, TUNICA VAGINALIS
et: Congenital incomplete closure of processus vaginalis; inflammation
sm: Pain mild to severe, usually when standing; progressive
sg: Pyriform mass in upper scrotum
cm: Infection; atrophy of testis; acute suppuration of tunica; chronicity
lb: Noninfected hydrocele: clear fluid

HYDROCELE, TUNICA VAGINALIS, TRAUMATIC
et: Direct violence; abnormal accumulation of fluid in tunica vaginalis, testis
sm: Pain; weakness; nausea; swelling in tunica vaginalis
sg: Cystic mass in tunica area, usually in upper part of scrotum; smooth, elastic, light transilluminated
cm: Chronicity
lb: Fluid usually hemorrhagic

HYPERHIDROSIS
et: Overactivity of sweat glands; obesity; anxiety
sg: Excessive sweating, predominant in axillae, genitocrural region, hands, feet; unexposed areas affected
cm: Maceration, fissuring; fungus infection often superimposed

HYPERVENTILATION SYNDROME
at: Alkalosis, Respiratory
et: Anxiety or hysterical state; deep breathing leading to excessive expiration of carbon dioxide

sm: Giddiness; faintness; agitation; tingling of toes, fingers, face; loss
     of consciousness
sg: Hyperventilation; muscle tremors; stupor
cm: Tetany

ILIOPECTINEAL BURSITIS

et: Excessive repetitive running
sm: Pain over anterior aspect of hip at about middle of inguinal liga-
     ment, possibly radiating down front of leg; disability
sg: Hip usually held in flexion, abduction, and external rotation; ten-
     derness
cm: Infection; persistent disability
pa: Irritation of bursa lying between iliopsoas and pelvis against ilio-
     pectineal eminence proximally and capsule of hip joint distally

ILIOPSOAS STRAIN

at: Groin Strain; Groin Pull
et: Excessive forcible contraction of iliopsoas with thigh fixed or
     forced into extension
sm: Pain in groin, especially in hip extension or rotation; disability in
     running or jumping
sg: Grade by degree of severity: thigh held in flexed adducted posi-
     tion; tenderness over anterior aspect of hip or near region of lesser
     trochanter along upper anteromedial aspect of thigh
cm: Recurrence; persistent disability
xr: May show avulsion of lesser trochanter

ILIUM FRACTURE, CREST AVULSION

et: Excessive forcible contraction of abdominal muscles while trunk
     is forced to contralateral side
sm: Severe pain along iliac crest, especially in attempt to straighten
     back; disability usually severe
sg: Walks in stooped position; usually extreme tenderness; palpable
     defect; crepitus; hematoma formation; ecchymosis
cm: Prolonged disability; recurrence
xr: Avulsion of iliac crest fragment with upward displacement

ILIUM FRACTURE, SPINE AVULSION

et: Anterosuperior spine pulled off by tensor fascia femoris and sar-
     torius during forcible running or jumping activity
sm: Local pain, especially on flexion or abduction of thigh; disability
sg: Local swelling and tenderness; fragment may be palpated
cm: Prolonged disability; recurrence
xr: Avulsion fracture with fragment displaced downward; anteropos-
     terior view of ilium helpful

ILIUM FRACTURE, WING

at: Ilium Crest Epiphysis Fracture-Separation
et: Direct violence; lateral crushing injury
sm: Local pain; disability
sg: Local swelling and tenderness; inability to bear weight or to abduct
     against resistance; deformity rarely palpable
xr: Fracture size variable; little or no tendency toward displacement
     of fragment

IMPETIGO

at: Impetigo Contagiosa
et: Infectious: usually staphylococcus, occasionally streptococcus; poor hygiene predisposing
sm: Pruritus
sg: Initially small, reddish macule; then, vesicle with thin top; later, serous and pustular ooze followed by crusting, possibly ulceration
cm: Prolonged course if untreated; acute nephritis (rare)

INFLUENZA

at: Flu; Grip; Catarrhal Fever
et: Infection: myxovirus; communicable
sm: Mild general prodrome or abrupt onset; headache, retroorbital pain; diffuse myalgia; abdominal pain; malaise; dizziness; chills; weakness; prostration; later, sneezing, rhinorrhea, dry throat
sg: Fever; relative bradycardia; flushed hot skin
cm: Pneumonia; secondary infection of paranasal sinuses, middle ear; prolonged debility; depression
xr: Chest normal or increase in vascular markings

INFRAPATELLAR BURSITIS

et: Direct blow over patellar ligament; excessive repetitive running or climbing
sm: Sharp pain with pendulum extension of knee; usually mild disability
sg: Tenderness over patellar ligament; fluctuant swelling on either side of patellar ligament; normal depression on either side of patellar ligament absent; limited active motion of knee

*INTERNAL CAROTID ARTERY OCCLUSION

et: Direct blow to neck; severe wrenching or twisting of neck with carotid artery caught by lateral process of atlas
sm: May be asymptomatic; may have paralysis and/or numbness of face and extremities, inability to speak, blindness in one eye. Symptoms transient if spasm, transient or permanent if thrombosis
sg: Absent carotid pulsation in neck; occasionally, pulsation transmitted from more proximal segment of artery despite occlusion; hemiplegia, hemihypesthesia, aphasia; contralateral pyramidal tract signs and hyperreflexia. Signs transient if spasm, transient or permanent if thrombosis
cm: Possible permanent neurologic disability, death
xr: Angiography demonstrates the site of occlusion or spasm of the artery
pa: Thrombosis or spasm occluding lumen

INTERTRIGO

at: Gaulding; Chafing
et: Mechanical friction producing abrasion where skin surfaces are in contact, such as groin, axillae; sweat contributory; obesity predisposing
sm: Pain; disability
sg: Erythema; mild maceration; may progress to marked hyperemia, denudation, erosion
cm: Infection; cellulitis

*INTRACEREBRAL HEMORRHAGE

at: Intracerebral Clot; Intracerebral Hematoma
et: Blow to head, particularly over temporal or occipital regions, causing extravasation of blood within the brain substance
sm: Headache; nausea, vomiting; progressive impairment of consciousness; progressive paresis with paralysis of extremities contralaterally
sg: Rise in blood pressure, drop in pulse rate; ipsilateral pupillary dilatation, aphasia, hemiparesis, hemiplegia, bilateral extensor plantar reflexes, increased tonus in the contralateral extremities; if occipital: ataxia, incoordination of extremities, nystagmus
cm: Permanent neurologic deficit; death
lb: Lumbar puncture may show elevated cerebrospinal fluid pressure, red blood cells, or increased protein content
xr: Angiography may show displacement of blood vessels, most frequently at the frontotemporal junction

ISCHIOGLUTEAL BURSITIS

at: Ischial Tuberosity Bursitis
et: Prolonged sitting on hard surface as in crew
sm: Pain over ischial tuberosity and radiating down back of thigh along hamstrings
sg: Local tenderness; pain elicited by active extension of hip or active flexion of knee, or passive flexion of hip or passive extension of knee (straight-leg raising)
cm: Suppuration; calcification of bursa
pa: Irritation of bursa lying between ischial tuberosity and gluteus maximus

ISCHIOPUBIC FRACTURE, RAMI

et: Crushing violence, either in lateral or anteroposterior direction
sm: Pain in pubic and perineal regions; inability to bear weight; may have symptoms of shock
sg: Local swelling and signs of trauma such as abrasions, contusions, lacerations; inability to lift leg on affected side; acute tenderness on palpation; deformity possible
cm: Rupture of urethra, urinary bladder; retroperitoneal hemorrhage
xr: Complete fractures of anterior pelvic ring; fragments displaced inward and override, or may be pushed backward; usually transverse or oblique, may be comminuted

ISCHIOPUBIC FRACTURE, RAMI AVULSION

et: Excessive forcible abduction of thigh
sm: Pain localized in ischiopubic region; disability
sg: Tenderness localized along subcutaneous edge of ischiopubic rami and to lateral side; pain elicited by passive abduction or on forced adduction of thigh
cm: Persistent disability; recurrence
xr: Avulsion of bony attachment of adductor muscles

ISCHIUM FRACTURE, INFERIOR RAMUS

et: Direct violence from front; lateral crushing injury or fall
sm: Pain localized over inferior ischial ramus; moderate disability
sg: Local tenderness and swelling; pain elicited by abduction or hyperextension of thigh
xr: Fracture of inferior ischial ramus; little tendency for displacement

ISCHIUM FRACTURE, SUPERIOR RAMUS
et: Direct violence from front; lateral crushing injury or fall
sm: Pain localized over superior ischial ramus; moderate disability
sg: Pain elicited by abduction or hyperextension of thigh
xr: Fracture of superior ischial ramus; little tendency for displacement

ISCHIUM FRACTURE, TUBEROSITY
et: Fall in sitting position
sm: Pain localized over ischial tuberosity
sg: Local tenderness; pain elicited by providing tension on hamstrings
xr: Fracture of ischial tuberosity

ISCHIUM FRACTURE, TUBEROSITY AVULSION
et: Excessive forcible action of long head of biceps femoris; forcible flexion of hip with knee extended, as in leading leg of hurdler
sm: Pain over ischial tuberosity; disability
sg: Local tenderness, crepitus, swelling; loose fragment may be palpable; pain elicited by contraction of biceps femoris or on straight-leg raising
cm: Painful nonunion; recurrence; extensive heterotopic ossification
xr: Avulsion fracture of ischial tuberosity; or, separation of epiphysis of ischial tuberosity

JOINT DISLOCATION
at: Joint Luxation
et: Direct or indirect violence to joint; sudden violent muscular contraction
sm: Local pain; disability
sg: Bones no longer in contact for normal articulation; deformity; most commonly shoulder, elbow, ankle, interphalangeal joints, acromioclavicular joint
cm: Injury to adjacent soft tissues; recurrence; stiffness; traumatic arthritis; aseptic necrosis (hip)
xr: Right angle view in two planes demonstrates total displacement
pa: Third degree ligamentous injury

JOINT LOOSE BODIES
at: Joint Mice
et: Osteochondritis dissecans; traumatic arthritis; osteochondral fracture; osteochondromatosis; knee most commonly affected joint
sm: Periodic aching; joint instability; recurrent locking of joint
sg: Loose body palpable through soft tissues when it lies in superficial part of joint; swelling; synovitis effusion; crepitus; muscle atrophy
cm: Progressive destruction of articular surfaces
xr: Loose bodies visualized; small opaque, unattached to bone; interposed between joint surfaces

JOINT SUBLUXATION
et: Direct or indirect trauma; sudden violent muscular contraction; congenital structural defect; reduction usually spontaneous
sm: Pain, disability; usually spontaneously relieved on resumption of normal position
sg: Partial displacement of articular surfaces; crepitus; most commonly shoulder, patella
cm: Dislocation; recurrence; weakness
pa: First or second degree ligamentous injury

KIDNEY CONTUSION
et: Direct blow; fall
sm: Acute pain in lumbar area, may be progressive; red urine
sg: Obvious distress; shock; tenderness in flank; sometimes associated with rib fracture
lb: Microscopic and gross hematuria
xr: Excretory urography
pa: Subcapsular hemorrhage

KIDNEY LACERATION
et: Direct blow; fall; sudden violent muscular action; diseased kidney, congenital anomaly vulnerable to slight trauma
sm: Acute pain in lumbar area, upper abdomen increasing with activity; nausea, vomiting; red urine
sg: Obvious distress; shock; tenderness, muscle spasm; ileus with abdominal distention; bulge in flank; tachycardia
cm: Severe shock; late effect: hypertension resulting from renal scarring
lb: Hematuria
xr: Excretory urography may demonstrate lesion

KNEE CALCIFICATION, MEDIAL COLLATERAL LIGAMENT
at: Pellegrini-Stieda Disease; Post-traumatic Para-articular Ossification
et: Reaction to medial collateral sprain, possibly with partial avulsion of adductor longus tendon; may follow localized blow at attachment of ligament
sm: Local pain; weakness of knee; variable disability
sg: Limitation of knee flexion; tenderness localized at medial femoral condyle; early: vague thickening of deep tissues; later: bony prominence palpable and frequently visible, usually firmly fixed
cm: Persistent disability
xr: Plaque of calcium along medial femoral condyle in vicinity of adductor tubercle, separated from tibia by band of radiolucency

KNEE CONTUSION
et: Direct blow; fall onto knee
sm: Local pain, stiffness
sg: Variable: local swelling, ecchymosis, perhaps overlying abrasion; tenderness; pain usually not elicited on movement; no instability, locking, effusion; early disappearance of signs and symptoms; suspicion of sprain or strain ruled out
cm: Aggravation by repeated contusions; bursitis, synovitis, tenosynovitis; ligamentous calcification
xr: Fracture, traumatic arthritis, and loose bodies ruled out

KNEE DISLOCATION
at: Tibiofemoral Dislocation
et: Direct violence to front of leg near knee; excessive forcible hyperextension; lateral leverage forces
sm: Severe pain; profound disability
sg: Obvious deformity; swelling; abnormal mobility at knee; shock
cm: Joint instability; damage to popliteal vessels and nerves; gangrene; traumatic arthritis; residual stiffness; irreducibility
xr: Tibia dislocated anteriorly, posteriorly, laterally, or medially, or may be rotated upon femur; associated fractures of upper end of

tibia
pa: Complete rupture of both cruciates, collateral and posterior ligaments

KNEE SPRAIN, ANTERIOR CRUCIATE LIGAMENT
et: Sudden forcible internal rotation of femur upon fixed tibia while knee is abducted and flexed; or, forcible hyperextension of knee and internal rotation of tibia on femur with associated rupture of medial collateral ligament; or, violent force from behind on leg with foot fixed (clipping) driving leg forward on thigh
sm: Pain; disability
sg: Grade by degree of severity: extreme swelling; marked instability; anterior drawer sign, tibia displacing forward on femur
cm: Chronic disability; traumatic arthritis
xr: May see avulsion of medial tubercle of tibial spine

KNEE SPRAIN, HYPEREXTENSION
et: Direct blow from front causing sudden forcible hyperextension of knee
sm: Pain behind knee, especially on passive extension; disability
sg: Grade by degree of severity: swelling; tenderness in popliteal region; ecchymosis; may have anteroposterior instability
cm: Persistent instability
xr: May show avulsion fracture of tibial spine and/or upper tibial posterior rim
pa: Posterior capsule stretched or torn; if severe, anterior cruciate ligament torn; posterior cruciate ligament also may be sprained

KNEE SPRAIN, LATERAL COLLATERAL LIGAMENT
at: Knee Sprain, Fibular Collateral Ligament; Knee Sprain, External Collateral Ligament
et: Forceful adduction of internally rotated knee
sm: Pain on lateral side of knee; weakness, instability; disability
sg: Grade by degree of severity: increase in adduction mobility on stress; tenderness; effusion; ecchymosis; hemarthrosis; palpable defect or thickness
cm: Peroneal nerve palsy; chronic instability
xr: Stress films show varus instability and/or avulsion of bony fragment from styloid process or fibula. CAUTION: Care must be taken not to injure peroneal nerve

KNEE SPRAIN, MEDIAL COLLATERAL LIGAMENT
at: Knee Sprain, Tibial Collateral Ligament; Knee Sprain, Internal Collateral Ligament
et: Excessive forcible eversion of foot and abduction of knee, usually with knee flexed and extensor mechanism relaxed
sm: Pain on medial side of knee; weakness, instability; disability
sg: Grade by degree of severity: increase in abduction mobility on stress; tenderness; effusion; ecchymosis; hemarthrosis; palpable defect or thickness
cm: Chronic instability; Pellegrini-Stieda disease; rotary instability
xr: Stress films show valgus instability and help rule out fracture-dislocation of distal femoral epiphysis

KNEE SPRAIN, POSTERIOR CRUCIATE LIGAMENT
et: Sudden forcible external rotation of femur with foot fixed while knee is adducted and flexed; or, forcible displacement of tibia backward on femur with knee flexed; or, fall onto flexed knee with

force received on upper end of tibia

sm: Pain on movement

sg: Grade by degree of severity: extreme swelling; loss of function; instability; ecchymosis; tibia tends to drop backward with knee flexed; pain elicited by backward pressure on tibia; posterior drawer sign

cm: Chronic disability; traumatic arthritis

LACERATION, SKIN

at: Cut; Gash; Cleat Wound

et: Tearing force; trauma to skin overlying bone

sm: Bleeding; pain

sg: Open wound; tenderness

cm: Infection, such as tetanus

LARYNGITIS, ACUTE

at: Hoarseness

et: Upper respiratory infection; overuse, misuse of voice; allergy; mechanical irritation from postnasal drip

sm: Dry, burning sensation; tickling to rawness

sg: Loss of voice; cough; fever; edema

cm: Obstruction of airway; chronicity

LARYNX INJURY

at: Clothesline Injury

et: Direct blow to larynx

sm: Pain in throat; difficulty in swallowing, inspiration; acute laryngospasm

sg: Local tenderness, swelling

cm: Hemorrhage; aspiration pneumonia; obstructed airway; permanent injury to vocal cords

lb: Laryngoscopy demonstrates ecchymosis, edema

LUMBOSACRAL SPRAIN

at: Low Back Pain

et: Abnormal forcible motion causing stress on lower back

sm: Variable degree of severity; pain on motion or stress; disability

sg: Muscle spasm; tenderness; limitation of motion

cm: Recurrence; chronicity

LUMBOSACRAL STRAIN

at: Lumbago (if chronic)

et: Trauma; excessive forcible stretching or repetitive use of muscles in lower back

sm: Variable degree of severity: pain on motion or muscle contraction; disability

sg: Muscle spasm; tenderness; occasionally swelling; limitation of motion

cm: Recurrence

LUNATE DISLOCATION

et: Forcible hyperextension and compression of wrist as in fall onto hand

sm: Local pain; disability

sg: Swelling on volar surface of wrist; hand held in slight flexion; tender depression palpable on dorsal surface; palpable mass deep in volar surface beneath flexor tendon

cm: Median nerve injury; traumatic arthritis; aseptic necrosis

xr: Lunate displaced volarward on lateral view; on anteroposterior view, lunate is manifested as abnormal triangular shadow overlapping capitate; navicular may be tilted forward

LYMPHADENITIS, ACUTE

et: Infection spread to lymph nodes from primary source of infection such as puncture wound, blister, callus, ingrown nail; usually staphylococcal or streptococcal

sm: Variable pain; chills; headache; malaise

sg: Palpable, enlarged lymph glands; tenderness; erythema; fever; tachycardia

cm: Abscess; septicemia; distant abscess

lb: Leukocytosis; positive culture from point of entry

pa: Inflamed lymph glands and adjacent tissue

LYMPHANGITIS, ACUTE

et: Secondary spread of infection from primary site through lymphatic vessels

sm: Chills; malaise; headache

sg: Fever; red linear streaks under skin, usually on extremity, spreading proximally from primary lesion

cm: Lymphadenitis; septicemia; distant abscess

lb: Positive culture at site of lesion

pa: Induration of lymph vessel and adjacent tissue

MANDIBLE FRACTURE

at: Fractured Jaw (Lower)

et: Trauma

sm: Local pain, especially on movement; inability to occlude teeth forcibly

sg: Swelling; local tenderness; crepitus; deviation to fracture side; restricted movement

cm: Osteomyelitis; malocclusion

xr: Fracture of alveolar process, body, condyloid process, epiphysis, or ramus

MAXILLA FRACTURE

et: Trauma

sm: Local pain

sg: Deformity; local tenderness, swelling; crepitus; subcutaneous emphysema

cm: Osteomyelitis

xr: Fracture of alveolar process, premaxilla, or zygomaxillary complex

MEDIAL COLLATERAL LIGAMENT BURSITIS (KNEE)

at: Medial Collateral Ligament Fibrositis; Tibial Collateral Ligament Bursitis

et: Repeated trauma

sm: Pain beneath medial collateral ligament; disability, especially after prolonged standing

sg: Tenderness; quadriceps atrophy; no joint instability; no derangement signs; mass possibly palpable (rare)

cm: Calcification in bursa

pa: Inflammation of bursa between longitudinal part of medial collateral ligament and capsule

MEDIAL COLLATERAL LIGAMENT SYNDROME (KNEE)

at: Tibial Collateral Ligament Syndrome

et: Postural strain: repeated mild valgus sprains of knee; displaced and deformed meniscus either stretches collateral ligament or continually irritates it or subjacent bursa

sm: No history of injury; sudden or insidious onset of pain over medial collateral ligament usually increased if weight bearing increased

sg: Pain aggravated by forced external rotation of tibia on femur or by bearing weight with knee in flexion

cm: Persistent disability

pa: Occult derangement of medial meniscus with marked thickening of its peripheral border in middle third, stretching of its anterior and posterior attachments, or evidence of old tears

MENISCUS, LATERAL, CYST

at: Semilunar Cartilage Cyst (lateral)

et: Mucoid degenerative process within meniscus; congenital defect in development of meniscus; ganglion-like structure resulting from trauma

sm: Continuous dull ache in knee; no locking

sg: Tense, slightly tender swelling which may progress to size of walnut; usually larger with knee in extension; may be found directly over joint line or near anterolateral aspect of fibular head or over lateral aspect of femoral condyle; seldom effusion

cm: Persistent disability

pa: Soft gelatinous material between peripheral surface of meniscus and synovial membrane

MENISCUS, LATERAL, DISCOID

et: Developmental anomaly

sm: Aching pain on lateral aspect of knee; weakness; no locking of knee

sg: Loud click felt and heard when knee is flexed or extended near limits of range of motion

cm: Persistent disability

xr: May show a widening of space between lateral condyles of femur and tibia

MENISCUS, LATERAL, TEAR

at: Torn Cartilage (lateral)

et: Forcible hyperflexion of knee; with foot fixed firmly upon ground, femur rotated outward upon tibia while knee is adducted and flexed as in squatting with heel against buttocks for long duration, duck waddle-type exercise; discoid may be predisposing

sm: Recurrent effusion, instability, disability, weakness, pain; snapping sensation upon full flexing or extending

sg: Effusion; tenderness along joint line, anterolaterally or posterolaterally; pain elicited at lateral side of knee by rotary stress; positive McMurray test with tibia internally rotated and adducted; audible and palpable click coming out of deep flexion; positive "grinding test" with patient prone

cm: Traumatic arthritis; meniscus cyst; concomitant ligamentous instability

xr: Radio-opaque arthography may demonstrate tear of meniscus

MENISCUS, MEDIAL, CYST

at: Semilunar Cartilage Cyst (medial)

et: Mucoid degenerative process within meniscus; congenital defect in development of meniscus; ganglion-type structure resulting from trauma

sm: Continuous dull ache in knee, worse after activity; no locking

sg: Tense, slightly tender swelling which may progress to size of walnut; usually larger with knee in extension; may be found at periphery in front of, through, or behind medial collateral ligament; may be mobile; seldom effusion

pa: Usually multiple, containing soft gelatinous material

MENISCUS, MEDIAL, TEAR

at: Torn Cartilage (medial)

et: Torsion injury; sudden forcible internal rotation of femur upon fixed tibia while knee is abducted and flexed

sm: Pain on function; locking, giving way, catching of knee; insecurity, weakness; inability to fully extend knee; snapping sensation at medial side of knee; disability

sg: Swelling; local tenderness; pain at anteromedial aspect of knee elicited on forced passive extension; limited range of extension motion; positive McMurray test with tibia externally rotated and abducted; audible, palpable click coming out of deep flexion; positive "grinding test" with patient prone; may palpate mass medially

cm: Traumatic arthritis; concomitant ligamentous instability

xr: Radio-opaque arthrography may show tear of meniscus

METACARPAL, FIRST, FRACTURE

at: Thumb Fracture

et: Violent axial compression on end of thumb; compression and forcible hyperextension as in fall onto abducted thumb

sm: Pain on movement of thumb; weakness

sg: Swelling, tenderness at base of thumb and in anatomical snuff box; false motion; crepitus

xr: Distal fragment drawn upward and backward with tendency to posterior and outward bowing; irregular transverse or oblique fracture, usually impacted; or, epiphyseal separation

METACARPAL FRACTURE, BASE

et: Direct blow against end of metacarpal; crushing blow over back of hand

sm: Local pain

sg: Local tenderness, swelling; deformity; crepitus

xr: Lateral view best

METACARPAL FRACTURE, NECK

at: Subcapital Fracture of Metacarpal; Boxer's Fracture

et: Direct violence as in striking of fist; most commonly 5th metacarpal

sm: Pain; disability

sg: Local swelling; tenderness over head and neck of metacarpal; head of metacarpal palpable in palm; shortening of metacarpal; knuckle of metacarpal less prominent

xr: Fracture demonstrated

METACARPAL FRACTURE, SHAFT

et: Direct violence; torsional force

sm: Local pain; disability

sg: Swelling; tenderness on palpation; deformity; crepitus; false motion

xr: Fracture demonstrated

METACARPOPHALANGEAL DISLOCATION

et: Forcible hyperextension of finger

sm: Pain; limitation of motion

sg: Obvious deformity; proximal phalanx displaced dorsally; slight flexion of proximal interphalangeal joint; head of metacarpal prominent in palm

xr: Base of phalanx rests dorsally upon neck of metacarpal

METACARPOPHALANGEAL, FIRST, DISLOCATION

et: Forcible hyperextension of thumb

sm: Pain; limitation of motion

sg: Obvious deformity; proximal phalanx displaced dorsally; flexion of interphalangeal joint above it; tenderness; swelling

cm: Recurrence; weakness; irreducibility

xr: Posterior dislocation of proximal phalanx of thumb with phalanx hyperextended on metacarpal, base of phalanx displaced backward and upward over head of metacarpal resting on neck or shaft of metacarpal

METACARPOPHALANGEAL, INDEX, VOLAR DISLOCATION

et: Forcible hyperextension of proximal phalanx of index finger

sm: Pain; disability

sg: Hyperextension of index metacarpophalangeal joint; slight flexion of interphalangeal joint above it; puckering of skin on volar aspect of joint; head of index metacarpal prominent in palm; ulnar deviation of index finger

cm: Irreducibility

xr: Metacarpal head displaced volarward and proximal phalanx dorsalward, resting on metacarpal head

pa: Deep transverse metacarpal ligament displaced dorsally with volar plate; metacarpal head further displaced volarward through palmar aponeurosis

METACARPOPHALANGEAL SPRAIN

et: Forcible hyperextension

sm: Pain; varying degree of instability

sg: Grade by degree of severity: local tenderness; pain elicited on motion

cm: Chronic instability

xr: May show avulsed fragments

METATARSAL, FIFTH, FRACTURE, BASE

et: Excessive forcible inversion and adduction of foot; sprain-fracture involving forceful pull of peroneus brevis tendon
sm: Local pain, especially on weight bearing; disability
sg: Tender, prominent swelling at base of 5th metatarsal; crepitus may be palpated; pain elicited by active eversion or passive inversion of foot
cm: Nonunion; prolonged disability
xr: Fracture line may pass through tip of tuberosity, base of tuberosity, or proximal end of bone

METATARSAL FRACTURE, BASE

et: Excessive forcible dorsiflexion of foot; leg hit from behind; sudden violent dorsiflexion at ankle
sm: Pain; disability in running and jumping
sg: Sharply localized tenderness; swelling; ecchymosis
cm: Persistent disability
xr: Fracture of base of metatarsal (usually several); may be comminuted, usually transverse or short oblique

METATARSAL FRACTURE, HEAD

et: Stubbing toe under foot; weight falling on foot
sm: Pain localized to metatarsophalangeal joint
sg: Localized swelling, tenderness, stiffness; deformity
cm: Traumatic arthritis
xr: Fracture of head of metatarsal, usually little displacement

METATARSAL FRACTURE, HEAD, CHONDRAL

et: Stubbing toe under foot
sm: Local pain; disability
sg: Local swelling, tenderness, stiffness; prominence and deformity; catching and clicking of joint
cm: Traumatic arthritis
xr: May be negative early; may resemble Freiberg's disease later

METATARSAL FRACTURE, HEAD, OSTEOCHONDRAL

et: Stubbing toe under foot
sm: Local pain; disability
sg: Local swelling, tenderness, and stiffness; prominence and deformity; catching and clicking
cm: Traumatic arthritis
xr: Osteochondral fracture of metatarsal head; may look like osteochondritis dissecans

METATARSAL FRACTURE, NECK

et: Stubbing toe under foot; weight falling on foot
sm: Local pain; disability in walking and running
sg: Local swelling and tenderness just proximal to joint; involved metatarsal head prominent in sole of foot; limited motion
cm: Metatarsalgia; malunion; nonunion
xr: Fracture of neck of metatarsal, usually with little displacement; may show plantar rotation of metatarsal head

METATARSAL FRACTURE, SHAFT

et: Crushing injury as in weight falling on foot
sm: Generalized pain of foot; disability
sg: Extensive swelling; pain elicited by axial pressure in line of shaft; crepitus demonstrated on gentle flexion and extension
cm: Prolonged disability; metatarsalgia; calluses; malunion
xr: Comminution; usually long or short oblique, transverse fracture; proximal end of distal fragment displaced into sole of foot; rotation of distal fragment

METATARSAL FRACTURE, SHAFT, FATIGUE

at: Metatarsal March Fracture; Metatarsal Stress Fracture
et: Excessive repetitive trauma as in walking or running long distances in heavy shoes, or on hard surfaces
sm: Pain along forefoot or arch, increasing on weight bearing or activity
sg: Local tenderness, especially on stretching plantar arch; increasing disability
xr: Early, usually negative; after three to four weeks, callus formation around metatarsal shaft or evidence of a simple transverse fracture across shaft

METATARSAL HEAD OSTEOCHONDRITIS

at: Freiberg's Disease; Koehler II Disease
et: Direct trauma as in jumping, kicking, stubbing toe, usually of 2nd toe
sm: Local pain, stiffness
sg: Elongated 2nd toe; local swelling; tenderness upon passive movement; may have palpable deformity
cm: Degenerative arthritis of metatarsophalangeal joint
xr: Early: irregular areas of condensation and rarefaction in epiphysis. Later: broadening and flattening of metatarsal head and shaft; S-shaped outline of articular surface; occasionally articular cartilage separated from underlying bone
pa: Aseptic necrosis

METATARSOPHALANGEAL DISLOCATION

et: Fall; stubbing toe under foot; weight falling on foot
sm: Pain, disability
sg: Deformity; toe maintained in abnormal position; swelling; ecchymosis
cm: Traumatic arthritis; irreducibility
xr: Metatarsophalangeal dislocation demonstrated

MIDTARSAL DISLOCATION

et: Crushing injury; torsion injury; fall from height
sm: Pain; disability
sg: Forefoot grossly displaced and foot shortened; head of talus, proximal borders of displaced anterior tarsal bones palpable; ankle motions not disturbed; malleoli intact; marked swelling of foot and ankle
cm: Traumatic arthritis; persistent disability
xr: Dislocation of talonavicular joint medially and calcaneocuboid joint laterally, separating anterior from posterior tarsal bones

MOLLUSCUM CONTAGIOSUM

at: Molluscum Epitheliale; Water Wart
et: Virus; auto-innoculation; mildly communicable
sm: Asymptomatic unless lesion inflamed
sg: Yellow to pink bulbous, sessile umbilicated papules on face, trunk, anogenital area; perhaps spontaneous involution
lb: Virus visualized by electron microscope or under darkfield

MONILIASIS, CUTANEOUS

et: Candida albicans
sm: Pruritus; burning pain; disability
sg: Well defined weeping, eroded lesion with scalloped border; collar of overhanging scales and intensely red base; satellite flaccid vesico pustules often present; usually found on groin, axillae, inframammary region, and between toes and webs of fingers
lb: Large quantities of budding cells and filaments of organism in scrapings seen under microscope; positive culture

MONONUCLEOSIS, INFECTIOUS

at: Glandular Fever
et: Unknown; possibly virus
sm: Variable, widespread manifestations: usually severe sore throat; course may be benign; headache; malaise; asthenia. Other less common manifestations: dysphagia, dyspnea from throat swelling; abdominal pain; skeletal muscle spasms and ascending type of paralysis; stiff neck; isolated palsies of face and extremities
sg: Variable: fever; inflammation; swelling of tonsils and pharyngeal tissues; enanthema of soft palate; phlegmonous exudate of tonsils; enlargement of anterior and posterior cervical glands; axillary and inguinal glands may be palpable; spleen and liver may be palpable; occasionally, fever and prostration present without anginal signs; mild jaundice; transient pink or brown maculopapular rash on trunk; other skin eruptions rare; diverse manifestations of neurological involvement
cm: Prolonged debility; Guillain-Barre syndrome; meningo-encephalitis; thrombocytopenia, hemolytic anemia (rare); rupture of spleen: sports participation contraindicated during active phase of illness and as long as evidence or suspicion of splenic enlargement exists
lb: Blood smear shows atypical lymphocytes. WBC: relative lymphocytosis; positive hetereophil agglutination test with specific absorption studies
xr: Flat plate of abdomen may reveal enlarged spleen; repeat x-ray indicated prior to return to sports
pa: Hyperplasia of lymphoid tissues; perivascular aggregates of normal and abnormal lymphocytes; focal lesions in myocardium, lungs, kidneys, skin, and central nervous system; enlarged soft spleen

MONTEGGIA FRACTURE

et: Indirect trauma producing excessive forcible pronation of forearm
sm: Pain; disability
sg: Deformity with anterior angulation of ulnar fragments associated with anterior dislocation of radial head; or, posterior angulation of ulna associated with posterior dislocation of radial head; elbow in partial flexion, midrotation; depression over posterior aspect of ulnar shaft; tenderness; swelling

cm: Permanent disability
xr: Fracture at junction of proximal and middle third of ulna with dislocation of head of radius, anteriorly or posteriorly

MOUTH, EXTRAORAL LACERATION
et: Direct blow; shearing force
sm: Local pain
sg: Local skin lesion; swelling; bleeding of lips, skin of dentofacial area, or vermillion border
cm: Infection, such as tetanus

MOUTH, INTRAORAL LACERATION
et: Inadvertent biting of tissue; external trauma; forceful displacement or damage by prosthetic or orthodontic appliance (rare)
sm: Local pain
sg: Local tenderness, swelling; bleeding of cheeks, gum, or tongue
cm: Infection

MYOSITIS OSSIFICANS, TRAUMATIC
et: Direct blow; contusion and hematoma involving muscle overlying bone; repeated irritation of injured area by unwise manipulation or too early activity; most common sites are anterior thigh (see charleyhorse) and brachialis muscle
sm: Local pain; disability
sg: Firm, immobile mass palpable deep in involved muscle subjacent to bone; tenderness; possible limitation of motion
cm: Misdiagnosis of malignant bone tumor; recurrence due to premature surgical removal
xr: Soft tissue mass early; later, characteristic lamination of ossification; eventually diminution of calcification or maturity of margins; finally, bony mass barely perceptible or takes form resembling exostosis
pa: Rapid deposition of osteoid bone; fibrous tissue replaces and separates striated muscle bundles; ossification of infiltrated blood along muscle origin on bone; (not fiber avulsion from periosteum; not subperiosteal hematoma; not calcification about traumatized joint or bone)

NAIL AVULSION
et: Sudden violence to nail as from foul tip in baseball, stubbing of toe; length of nail a factor
sm: Sharp pain; disability
sg: Bleeding; nail loose or missing; tenderness
cm: Low-grade infection; disturbance in nail regrowth

NAIL, SUBUNGUAL HEMATOMA
et: Direct blow to nail
sm: Progressive intense throbbing pain; disability
sg: Blue, cyanotic discoloration
cm: Loss of nail; infection

NAIL, TOE, INGROWN
at: Unguis Incarnatus
et: Mechanical irritation as from tight shoes; poor cutting of nail; local trauma

sm: Pain, especially on activity; variable disability
sg: Edge of nail imbedded in skin; tenderness; erythema; swelling
cm: Infection; local suppuration

NERVE CONTUSION
at: Nerve Compression; Traumatic Neuritis; Pinched Nerve
et: Direct trauma, perhaps recurrent trauma, causing swelling of nerve under a ligament; may be in association with fracture of an extremity
sm: Dermatomal numbness and paresthesia and/or weakness in the muscles involved
sg: Tenderness over site of contusion; hypalgesia in dermatome and weakness or paralysis of muscles supplied by the nerve
cm: Possible permanent loss of sensation and motor function of muscles supplied by nerve
lb: EMG may show positive findings three weeks after nerve injury; possible loss of nerve conduction time

NEURITIS
at: Inflamed Nerve
et: Infection; diabetes mellitus; other constitutional disorders
sm: Pain over course of nerve, increasing at night; numbness or pain aggravated by movement; weakness
sg: Possible hyperesthesia in dermatome
cm: Contractures; muscle fibrosis; paralysis; atrophy of muscles and nerves involved; possible inflammatory cell reaction

NEURODERMATITIS, LOCALIZED
at: Lichen Simplex, Chronic
et: Unknown; psychogenic factors
sm: Severe, persisting paroxysmal pruritus
sg: Circumscribed scaling patch with sharp margins; dry brown or yellow, solitary or symmetrical eruptions on anterolateral aspects of leg, proximal dorsal area of forearm, sacrococcygeal area, or nuchal region

NOSE CONTUSION
et: Direct blow to nose
sm: Variable pain; epistaxis; local swelling sensation, perhaps impaired breathing
sg: Swelling; ecchymosis; evidence of epistaxis; may have deformity from laterally displaced nasal cartilage; tenderness
cm: Deviated septum
xr: Nose fracture ruled out; other facial fracture may be present

NOSE FRACTURE
et: Direct blow
sm: Pain; impaired breathing; epistaxis
sg: Obvious deformity; evidence of epistaxis; septum displacement possible; swelling with obstruction of nasal passage(s); later: swelling and ecchymosis of eyelid, subconjunctival hemorrhage; perhaps local anesthesia and lost sense of smell; rhinorrhea if cribiform plate fracture
cm: Permanent deformity and nasal obstruction; infection
xr: Demonstrates site and extent of fracture; depressed fracture if from frontal blow, laterally displaced fracture if from lateral blow

OLECRANON BURSITIS

at: Water on Elbow; Student Elbow
et: Repeated friction; trauma; infection; may be associated with gout
sm: Pain; moderate disability
sg: Tenderness; swelling; limited motion in severe cases
cm: Chronicity
xr: May show calcification of bursa

ORBIT BLOWOUT FRACTURE

et: Trauma producing sudden increase in intraorbital pressure; blow to soft tissues in orbital area from fist or object
sm: Diplopia; anesthesia or hypesthesia of cheek along distribution of infraorbital nerve; enophthalmos; eye muscle imbalance
sg: Ecchymosis; swelling; subconjunctival hemorrhage; hyphema; inability of eye to rotate upward in normal range
cm: Permanent visual disturbances, diplopia if untreated; glaucoma; cataract formation
xr: Waters' view shows fracture in floor of orbit and increased density in antrum
pa: Downward displacement of orbital floor with extrusion of orbital soft tissue into maxillary sinus

ORCHITIS, TRAUMATIC

et: Trauma to testis
sm: Sudden pain in testis, radiating to inguinal canal; nausea, vomiting
sg: Ecchymosis of scrotal area; swollen, tense, tender testis, may be fluctuant
cm: Atrophy of testis; sterility

OSGOOD-SCHLATTER'S DISEASE

at: Tibial Tubercle Osteochondrosis; Tibial Tubercle Apophysitis
et: Unknown; trauma; osteochondritis; excessive forcible pull of patellar tendon on tibial tubercle; avulsion of superficial portion of tibial tubercle epiphysis; limited to early adolescence
sm: Pain over tibial tubercle, increasing during strenuous activity or on kneeling; disability
sg: Enlargement of tibial tubercle; local tenderness; possibly distention and enlargement of infrapatellar bursa
cm: Loose bodies formed in or under patellar tendon; recurrence until epiphysis closes; symptoms may persist into adulthood
xr: Enlargement and sometimes fragmentation of tibial tubercle; may be a sequestrated fragment; sclerosis; swelling of soft tissues anterior to insertion of patellar tendon

OSTEOCHONDRITIS DISSECANS

et: Unknown; impairment of blood supply to affected segment of bone by thrombosis of an end artery; injury predisposing
sm: Knee most common site; discomfort or pain after exercise; chronic, nonspecific, intermittent swelling; recurrent sudden locking and instability
sg: Effusion; muscle atrophy; crepitus; limited movement; locking
cm: Traumatic arthritis
xr: Clear-cut crescentic excavation of bone at articular surface; at first, cavity occupied by separating bone fragment; later, cavity may be empty, and a loose body seen elsewhere in joint; tangential

view best

pa: Local necrosis of segment of articular surface on bone and of overlying articular cartilage

OSTEOCHONDROMA

et: Unknown; appears primarily between ages 10-25 years
sm: Slight discomfort in adjacent joint
sg: Circumscribed hard swelling near a joint
cm: Pathological fracture
lb: Benign bone tumor
xr: Osseous base or pedicle of normal bone density springing directly from cortex of underlying bone and capped by an expanded area of cartilage showing irregular calcification; typically situated near ends of long bones

OSTEOCHONDROMATOSIS, SYNOVIAL

et: Unknown; trauma (secondary); benign metaplastic error of synovial cells
sm: Increasingly severe local pain; intermittent pain; locking; instability
sg: Intermittent swelling; limitation of motion; tenderness; firm, irregular feeling; crepitus
cm: Traumatic arthritis; postsurgical recurrence; chondrosarcoma (rare)
xr: Spotty calcific changes throughout joint; intra-articular loose bodies
pa: Benign, tumorous multifocal chondro-osseous metaplastic proliferation involving subsynovial connective tissue; thickened synovial membrane

OSTEOGENIC SARCOMA

et: Unknown; occurs primarily during adolescence
sm: Gradually increasing local pain
sg: Gradually increasing local swelling; diffuse, firm thickening near end of bone; overlying skin warm
cm: Pathological fracture; malignancy, metastasis to lung or other bones
xr: Irregular destruction of metaphysis; later, cortex appears to have been burst open; usually, evidence of new bone formation under corners of raised periosteum
pa: Arising from primitive osteoblasts, destruction of bone substance and eventual bursting into surrounding tissue

OSTEOID OSTEOMA

et: Unknown; benign tumor or infective lesion hypothesized
sm: Severe deep boring pain, poorly localized, especially at night; relief by salicylates diagnostic
sg: Thickening and local tenderness at site of lesion
xr: Local sclerotic thickening of shaft with small central area of rarefaction which may be visible only on laminograms; usually found in cortex of long bone but occasionally in cancellous bone

OSTEOMYELITIS, ACUTE

at: Bone Infection, Acute
et: Pyogenic organisms; hematogenous; secondary to acute local infection, compound fracture or other trauma, penetrating wound
sm: History of recent contusion or other bone injury; sudden pain in

affected bone; malaise; prostration; chills

sg: Fever; acute tenderness; erythema; edema; pain elicited on movement of limb

cm: Chronicity; deep seated infection around sequestra in depths of bone; may break through into contiguous joint

lb: Leukocytosis; increased sedimentation rate; positive culture

xr: May be negative early; later, rarefied, mottled medulla; clearly defined new bone jointed to cortex; sequestra necrotic bone cast off

pa: Local necrosis in bone marrow near end of shaft soon spreads along marrow cavity; exudate may break through surface and form subperiosteal abscess

OVARIAN HEMORRHAGE

at: Mittelschmerz

et: Graafian follicle rupture, usually midway between menses

sm: Lower abdominal pain on either side; may resemble appendicitis

sg: Abdominal tenderness; may get adnexal mass if severe

cm: Severe hemorrhage (rare)

lb: Usually mild leukocytosis; lowered hemoglobin and hematocrit with extensive hemorrhage

PARONYCHIA

et: Infection; pulling on hangnail; other trauma contributory

sm: Pain at site of infection between nail and cuticle

sg: Tenderness, erythema; purulent discharge

cm: Subungual abscess; extension of infection; septicemia

lb: Positive culture

PATELLA CHONDROMALACIA

et: Unknown; trauma; may be secondary to recurrent subluxation

sm: Discomfort, especially on flexion or extension of knee against resistance; catching, transient locking, instability, weakness of knee

sg: Tenderness on palpating deep surface of patella after lateral displacement; fine crepitus; effusion

cm: Traumatic arthritis; loose bodies in knee joint

xr: Early: negative. Late: diminished space between back of patella and femur; lipping of patella; rarefaction or condensation of adjacent bone

pa: Articular cartilage of patella roughened and fibrillated

PATELLA DISLOCATION, ACUTE

et: Violence against medial aspect of patella from forcible rotation of femur on fixed tibia, lateral rotation of tibia on fixed femur

sm: Severe pain; disability

sg: May reduce spontaneously by straightening knee; hemarthrosis; swelling; tenderness along superomedial border; tibia in position of abduction; muscle spasm; palpable defect along medial border of patella

cm: Recurrent dislocation; osteochondral fracture of patella or lateral femoral condyle; chondromalacia of patella

xr: Unreduced: patella rotated through 90° and articular surface lies in contact with lateral side of lateral femoral condyle. Reduced: increased tibiofemoral angle; shallow patellar groove on silhouette view; arthrogram shows rupture of medial capsule; fragmentation if avulsion of retinaculum

PATELLA DISLOCATION, RECURRENT

et: Predisposing bony architecture; high-riding patella, shallow intercondylar groove, genu valgum; excessive forcible external rotation
of tibia; weakness of vastus medialis; trauma to medial aspect of
knee

sm: Severe sudden pain, disability

sg: Deformity if patella still displaced; Postreduction: atrophy of
vastus medialis; patellar tendon and medial capsule lax; patella
almost dislocates laterally by simple pressure; flexion of knee displaces patella laterally; synovial thickening

cm: Chondromalacia of patella; osteochondral fracture of patella,
lateral femoral condyle; traumatic arthritis

xr: Lateral femoral condyle underdeveloped; patella displaced laterally;
osteochondral fracture; medial half of patella underdeveloped

PATELLA FRACTURE

at: Fractured Kneecap

et: Indirect violence as in snapping of patella over condyles from force
applied to semiflexed knee; sudden violent contraction of quadriceps mechanism; jumping or fall from height; direct blow

sm: Pain; disability

sg: Hemarthrosis; swelling; ecchymosis; sulcus palpated between fractured segments; false motion without crepitus

cm: Nonunion; residual stiffness; traumatic arthritis

lb: Aspiration shows fat particles in blood

xr: Transverse fracture; comminution; variable displacement; loose
fragments displaced into knee joint

PATELLA FRACTURE, AVULSION, INFERIOR POLE

et: Sudden forcible hyperextension or flexion of knee

sm: Pain localized to inferior pole of patella; disability

sg: Local tenderness, swelling; crepitus; defect may be palpable; pain
elicited by active extension and passive flexion

cm: Atrophy of quadriceps femoris

xr: Avulsion fracture of inferior pole of patella; main fragment displaced upward

PATELLA FRACTURE, AVULSION, SUPERIOR POLE

et: Sudden forcible extension or flexion of knee

sm: Pain localized to superior pole of patella; disability

sg: Local tenderness and swelling; crepitus; defect may be palpable;
pain elicited by active extension and passive flexion

cm: Atrophy of quadriceps femoris

xr: Avulsion fracture of superior pole of patella; small fragment displaced upward

PATELLA FRACTURE, CHONDRAL

et: Fall onto flexed knee; recurrent subluxational forces

sm: Persistent pain; locking or catching of knee; disability

sg: Swelling; hemarthrosis; tenderness, especially on rubbing patella
against condylar groove with knee in complete extension; pain
elicited by flexion and extension of knee against resistance

cm: Traumatic arthritis; residual joint dysfunction; persistent disability

xr: Ordinary films negative; radio-opaque arthrography may show

78

radiolucent defect in knee
pa: Contusion, fissuring of articular cartilage; complete chondral fracture with piece of cartilage separated from bone

PATELLA FRACTURE, LATERAL MARGINAL

et: Direct violence applied to periphery of patella, forcing patella against lateral condyle of femur

sm: Pain on lateral aspect of patella, especially with movement through range of motion; later, pain in retropatellar region during activity; disability

sg: Local swelling; tenderness; crepitus; effusion

cm: Nonunion; traumatic arthritis

xr: Vertical or longitudinal fracture, not to be confused with bipartite patella; minimal displacement; axial view helpful

PATELLA FRACTURE, MEDIAL TANGENTIAL

et: Complication of acute traumatic or recurrent subluxation or dislocation of patella; the quadriceps, contracting to recover position exerts tangential force, shearing off portion of patellar articular cartilage plus a wedge-shaped fragment of underlying cancellous tissue from inframedial margin of articular surface

sm: History of recent subluxation or dislocation of patella; retropatellar pain; locking; disability

sg: Retropatellar tenderness; effusion; limitation of motion

cm: Traumatic arthritis; persistent disability

xr: Osteochondral fragment displaced into joint; purely chondral fragment may be detected by radio-opaque arthrograph; axial radiograph shows shallow intercondylar groove, irregularity of medial aspect of patella

PATELLA FRACTURE, OSTEOCHONDRAL

et: Fall upon flexed knee; recurrent subluxational force

sm: Persistent pain; locking, catching; disability

sg: Swelling; hemarthrosis; tenderness, particularly on rubbing patella against condylar groove with knee in full extension; pain elicited by flexion and extension of knee against resistance

cm: Traumatic arthritis; residual joint dysfunction

lb: Aspiration shows fat particles in blood

xr: Osteochondral fragment in knee joint; oblique films and skyline view helpful; defect of articular surface of patella

PATELLA OSTEOCHONDRITIS

et: Vigorous activity as in running and jumping on hard surfaces, or running up and down hills; occurs primarily during ages 10-14

sm: Mild pain around patella; may be bilateral; symptoms aggravated by activity

sg: Tenderness and swelling located to inferior (Larsen-Johansson's Disease) or superior pole; leg extension against resistance may produce pain

cm: Disability

xr: Early: negative. Later: fragmentation of inferior or superior pole; may be some calcification present in patellar tendon

pa: Hemorrhage and degenerative changes in patellar ligament or quadriceps tendon

PATELLA OSTEOCHONDRITIS DISSECANS

et: Trauma; impingement of articular surfaces; underlying constitutional disorder

sm: Vague pain relieved by rest; knee gives way during activity; sensation of loose bodies; intermittent disability

sg: Effusion; loose body palpated; synovial thickening; muscle atrophy; crepitus; tenderness; limitation of motion

cm: Persistent disability; traumatic arthritis

xr: Best seen on lateral and/or skyline views; crescentic cavity in patella with separating of fragment in situ; later, loose body may be seen elsewhere in joint

PATELLA SUBLUXATION, ACUTE

et: Blow against medial aspect of patella; medial rotation of femur on fixed tibia or lateral rotation of tibia on fixed femur combined with increased lateral mobility of patella; predisposing factors include genu valgum, shallow patella groove, tendon attachment to lateral side of tibia midline, excessive external rotation of tibia

sm: Severe pain; loss of motion and function

sg: May reduce spontaneously on straightening knee; hemarthrosis; swelling; tenderness along superomedial border of bone; semiflexion of knee shows abnormal position of patella; extreme apprehension of examiner's palpation; spasm

cm: Recurrent subluxation of patella; osteochondral fracture of patella or lateral femoral condyle; chondromalacia of patella

xr: Patella lies on lateral border of lateral condyle; increased tibiofemoral angle; silhouette view demonstrates shallow patellar groove

PATELLA SUBLUXATION, RECURRENT

et: Abnormally high patella; shallow intercondylar groove; genu valgum; excessive external rotation of tibia; weakness of vastus medialis; relatively minor blow to medial side of patella

sm: Insecurity; recurrent attacks of synovial effusion; instability; pain

sg: Tenderness over anteromedial aspect of knee; wasting of vastus medialis; lax patellar tendon and medial capsule; increased lateral mobility of patella compared to other side; apprehension of examiner's attempt to laterally displace patella; synovial thickening; knee flexion displaces patella laterally

cm: Chondromalacia of patella; osteochondral fracture of patella or lateral femoral condyle; traumatic arthritis

xr: Lateral femoral condyle underdeveloped; patella located at higher and more lateral level than normal; medial half of patella underdeveloped

PATELLAR TENDON STRAIN

et: Repeated jumping; fall from height; stumbling

sm: Inability to extend knee; pain localized over front of knee

sg: Grade by degree of severity: hemarthrosis; general tenderness; subcutaneous swelling at site of tendon injury just below patella; patella displaced upward intact and not tender; definite impression in tissues palpable below patella

cm: Chronic weakness

xr: Small fragment of bone may be avulsed from lower pole of patella

PEDICULOSIS PUBIS

at: Crabs
et: Irritation from saliva, excreta of crab louse; louse transmitted by body contact or close proximity
sm: Pruritus of pubis, waist, and contiguous hairy areas; may extend to axilla and eye brows
sg: Lice, ova, macroscopically visible in involved areas; small, red papules; excoriations; crusting after scratching; brownish pigmentation in cases of long duration
cm: Secondary infection
lb: Identification of parasite

PELVIS FRACTURE

et: Fall from height; direct blow
sm: Pain, especially on motion or weight bearing; disability
sg: Local swelling; ecchymosis; tenderness; pain elicited by strong pelvic compression
cm: Rupture of viscera; rupture of rectum, vagina; retroperitoneal hemorrhage; neural damage; shock; deformity; thrombophlebitis
xr: Fracture of one or more portions of pelvic ring

PEPTIC ULCER SYNDROME

et: Inability of gastrointestinal mucosa to withstand proteolytic action of acid gastric juice; vascular states related to stasis, congestion; emotional stress producing hyperacidity, hypermotility; apparent relationship to adrenal cortical activity, administration of steroids
sm: Epigastric pain varying with site, size of lesion; time relationship to ingestion of food; nocturnal pain; nausea, vomiting
sg: Aggravation of symptoms by spicy foods, alcohol, nicotine; relieved by milk and alkalis; local tenderness
cm: Perforation; hemorrhage; obstruction; fistula; anemia
lb: Gastric analysis demonstrates increased gastric acidity with extreme response to histamine; fluoroscopy may show abnormal peristalsis with delayed gastric emptying
xr: Barium administration may reveal niche or crater in stomach or duodenum

PERILUNAR DISLOCATION

at: Retrolunar Dislocation
et: Excessive forcible hyperextension of wrist as in fall onto outstretched hand
sm: Wrist pain; median nerve paresthesias; disability
sg: Obvious deformity; swelling; tenderness over wrist; increased diameter of wrist; crepitus
cm: Traumatic arthritis; carpal tunnel syndrome; disability if unreduced
xr: Hand and carpal bones dislocated backward leaving lunate bone in position; anteroposterior view may show widened space between navicular and lunate with abnormal triangular appearance of lunate partly overlapping capitate; lateral view shows navicular dislocated posteriorly

PERIODONTITIS

at: Pyorrhea
et: Local causes: calculus, food impaction, Vincent's infection, broad contact points. Systemic causes: diabetes, blood dyscrasias, dilantin sodium therapy for epilepsy

sm: Local pain; malaise; bleeding
sg: Redness, swelling; bleeding; local tenderness; pain elicited by percussion of adjacent tooth
cm: Parietal abscess
pa: Inflammation, hypoplasia of epithelium and connective tissue; loss of alveolar bone

PERIOSTITIS, TRAUMATIC

at: Bone Bruise; Stone Bruise
et: Direct blow to bone; muscle strain at attachment to bone; infection invading subperiosteal region; heel is most common site
sm: Local pain; varying disability
sg: Subperiosteal hematoma may be palpable; exquisite local tenderness; erythema; muscle spasm
cm: Permanent osseous thickening; prolonged disability
lb: Aspiration of subperiosteal hematoma blood or clear fluid
xr: Formation of new lamellae of bone parallel to surface; new osseous density conforming to density of cortex; rarefaction absent
pa: Inflammation of periosteum covering bone

PERONEAL NERVE CONTUSION

et: Direct blow over head of fibula
sm: Pain over upper fibular region along lateral aspect of leg; tingling sensation down lateral side of leg and dorsum of foot; disability
sg: Paresthesia or hypesthesia of dorsum of foot and outer side of leg; foot drop, inability to dorsiflex foot or extend toes; local tenderness
cm: Permanent foot drop; equinus contracture of ankle

PERONEAL SPASTIC FLATFOOT

et: Unknown
sm: Pain in foot appearing in adolescence, usually after prolonged use; relieved at rest; disability
sg: Valgus deformity at subtalar and midtarsal joints; intertarsal joint movements limited and distorted; spasm of peroneal muscles precipitated by overuse
cm: Persistent disability; traumatic arthritis
xr: Talus fuses to calcaneus on their medial surfaces by bridge of bone; or a calcaneonavicular bar, or, one of several different intertarsal fusions may be present

PERONEAL TENDON DISLOCATION, ACUTE

et: Blow back of lateral malleolus while peroneal tendons are taut in dorsiflexion or eversion of foot; shallow peroneal groove predisposing; torn peroneal retinaculum; usually associated with other ankle injuries
sm: Local pain; disability
sg: Tendon displaced over lateral malleolus; usually spontaneous reduction; local tenderness and swelling; tendons not displaceable; local pain elicited by passive inversion of foot
cm: Tenosynovitis of peroneal tendons; recurrence; persistent disability
xr: May see some soft tissue calcification along lateral malleolus

PERONEAL TENDON DISLOCATION, RECURRENT

et: Congenitally shallow peroneal groove; untreated acute episode of dislocation; blow back of lateral malleolus while tendons are taut in dorsiflexion or eversion of foot sm: Recurrent sensation of tendon slipping out of place with sharp pain accompanying; spontaneous reduction relieves sensation; ankle weakness; recurrent disability

sg: Active eversion with tendons produces dislocation with snapping; shallow peroneal groove with thickening of peroneal retinaculum; local tenderness and swelling

cm: Tenosynovitis of peroneal tendons; persistent disability

PERONEAL TENOSYNOVITIS

et: Excessive forcible use of peroneal tendons; running with foot everted; recurrent tendon dislocation

sm: Pain localized behind lateral malleolus and along lateral aspect of foot; disability

sg: Local tenderness, swelling, erythema, crepitus; pain elicited by passive inversion and active eversion of foot

cm: Persistent or recurring disability

PHARYNGITIS, ACUTE

at: Sore Throat

et: Exudative and nonexudative types of infection; streptococcus, staphylococcus, other bacteria, virus

sm: Burning pain, dryness, sensation of lump in throat; cough; dysphagia; malaise; chills; headache

sg: Red, swollen pharyngeal mucosa; possibly exudate; cervical lymphadenopathy; possibly high fever

cm: Pharyngeal abscess; rheumatic fever (if streptococcal)

lb: Leukocytosis; culture identification of organism

PILONIDAL CYST, INFECTED

at: Pilonidal Sinus, Infected

et: Inflamed congenital remnant of primitive neuroectodermal canal overlying coccyx or sacral area; aggravated by trauma, superimposed infection

sm: Pain, swelling at base of spine

sg: Inflamed tender mass; draining, suppurative sinus; protruding hairs

cm: Local spread of infection with formation of serpiginous tracts; postsurgical recurrence

pa: Invagination of epithelium; ingrowth of hair; downgrowth of surface epithelium

PITYRIASIS ROSEA

et: Unknown; may be viral, noncommunicable; mild course; recurrence uncommon

sm: Pruritus; malaise; psychic disturbance

sg: Early: single annular lesion (herald patch) usually on trunk; generalized eruption follows in one week; oval lesions with salmon-colored slightly raised scaling border; usually on neck, trunk, upper portion of extremities with long axes along the lines of cleavage

pa: Mild to moderate nonspecific dermal inflammation with lymphocytic infiltration

PLANTAR FASCIITIS

et: Unknown; may be traumatic or postural as in arch sprain

sm: Pain beneath anteromedial part of calcaneum on standing or walk-

ing which may extend forward into sole
sg: Marked tenderness over site of attachment of plantar fascia to calcaneum
xr: May find sharp heel spur projecting forward from plantar aspect of calcaneal tuberosity
pa: Inflammation of fascia and soft connective tissue at site of plantar fascia attachment on inferior aspect of calcaneal tuberosity

PLANTAR NEUROMA
at: Morton's Toe; Morton's Metatarsalgia
et: Neuroma of plantar nerve at point where medial and lateral branches join and then separate to pass to adjacent sides of 3rd and 4th toes; thickening where "X" is formed subject to trauma when impinged between metatarsal heads; relaxation of intermetatarsal ligaments which permits splaying of forefoot contributory
sm: Intermittent, excruciating pain in lateral aspect of forefoot frequently relieved by removal of shoe; disability
sg: Exquisite tenderness between 3rd and 4th metatarsal heads on pressure in plantar surface of web, or by rolling heads across each other; small tender mass of nerve and fibrous tissue may be palpable

PLANTAR WART
at: Verruca Plantaris
et: Virus infection; susceptibility of host predisposing factor; often confused with callus
sm: Local pain as on walking
sg: Occurs anywhere on plantar surface while calluses show only on pressure points; do not project beyond skin surface; punctate areas of bleeding; distinct demarcation of edge; local tenderness; mosaic type characterized by numerous satellites refractory to treatment
cm: May spread, especially on contiguous surfaces; communicable through direct or indirect contact
pa: Simple papilloma growing outward from basal layers of skin with thickening of skin

PLANTARIS STRAIN
et: Forcible stretch as in running, jumping; excessive unaccustomed activity
sm: Pain in calf on running and jumping; sudden sharp pain deep in calf, if severe; disability
sg: Grade by degree of severity: tenderness about ten inches below knee on lateral side or in middle; nodule may be palpable in calf; pain elicited by dorsiflexing foot; plantarflexion unaffected
cm: Calcification of plantaris; thrombophlebitis

PNEUMONIA, ACUTE
et: Infection: virus; pneumococcus; Friedlaender bacillus; streptococcus; staphylococcus; hemophilus influenzae
sm: Malaise; chills; cough; expectoration; bloody sputum; shortness of breath; pleuritic pain; prostration
sg: Crepitant rales; bronchial breath-sounds; sputum turbid, later purulent, blood-tinged; possible high fever; dyspnea; cyanosis; pleural frictional rub; if virus, usually dry, nonproductive cough
cm: Empyema; abscess; purulent pericarditis; pleural thickening
lb: Identification of organism by culture; if bacteria, leukocytosis; if

viral, white blood cell decreased or normal with lymphocytosis
xr: Increased density of involved segment or lobe of lung; if lobar, patchy infiltration; if bronchal, diffuse increase

PNEUMOTHORAX, SPONTANEOUS
at: Collapsed Lung (Spontaneous)
et: Ruptured emphysematous or subpleural bleb; idiopathic; tuberculosis or fungal infection to be ruled out
sm: Abrupt onset of moderate to severe pain in chest or shoulder; shortness of breath; occasionally prostration
sg: Diminished chest excursion on affected side; hyperresonance with decreased or absent tactile fremitus and breath sounds; shock (rare)
cm: Hemothorax; serious respiratory disturbance; continued bleeding; infection
xr: Outline of collapsed lung, best visualized with expiration; mediastinum may shift to opposite side; fluid level visualized in pleural space

PNEUMOTHORAX, TRAUMATIC
at: Collapsed Lung (Traumatic)
et: Direct, sharp blow in back of chest area causing tear of pleura at its attachment to large bronchi; penetrating wound
sm: Pain in chest; shortness of breath on exertion; prostration in severe cases, especially in penetrating wound
sg: Diminished chest excursion on affected side; hyperresonance with decreased or absent tactile fremitus and breath sounds; tracheal shift; tachycardia; shock in severe cases
cm: Hemothorax; serious respiratory disturbances; continual bleeding; infection
xr: Outline of collapsed lung, best visualized with expiration; fluid level visualized in pleural space

POPLITEAL CYST
at: Baker's Cyst; Popliteal Bursitis; Medial Gastrocnemius Bursitis
et: Posterior damage to medial meniscus; hernia of semitendinosus sheath; synovial hernia at back of knee from defect or degeneration of posterior capsule; bursa wall expanded posteriorly between medial head of gastrocnemius and semitendinosus tendon
sm: Varying periods of chronic, aching type of pain in back of knee
sg: Periodic evidence of large soft tissue in popliteal space
cm: Contents of bursal sac may discharge into knee, causing synovitis
xr: Radio-opaque arthrography with dye extravasation shows soft tissue mass in popliteal region

POPLITEUS TENDON AVULSION
et: Forcible twisting of knee
sm: Pain over posterolateral aspect of knee; pain may be referred to lateral aspect of lateral femoral condyle and posterior upper calf; disability
sg: Local tenderness and swelling; pain elicited by forced extension and internal rotation of knee
cm: Persistent disability
xr: May show avulsion of fragment of bone from lateral aspect of lateral femoral condyle; radio-opaque arthrography may show unusual extravasation of dye into and down popliteal recess

85

POSTERIOR TIBIAL TENDON DISLOCATION

et: Violent twist of ankle such as from falling into hole; direct blow on extended leg with foot either in everted position or propped on object

sm: Severe pain in ankle and leg; disability

sg: Tendon rides out over medial malleolus; restricted ankle motion; swelling; tenderness behind medial malleolus

cm: Recurrence; persistent disability

xr: Oblique films may show soft tissue calcification adjacent to and behind medial malleolus

POSTERIOR TIBIAL TENDON TENOSYNOVITIS

et: Excessive forcible use of posterior tibial tendon as in running with foot inverted

sm: Pain localized behind medial malleolus; disability

sg: Tenderness, swelling, erythema, crepitus behind medial malleolus and along medial aspect of foot; pain elicited by active inversion and passive eversion of foot

cm: Recurrence; persistent disability

PREPATELLAR BURSITIS

at: Housemaid's Knee

et: Direct trauma; fall on flexed knee; friction as in kneeling position in wrestling

sm: Local pain; moderate disability

sg: Tenderness, erythema, and inflammation over knee; crepitus; effusion; tense and hot swelling over patella; ordinary motion is pain free but flexion to point of skin tension elicits pain; numerous palpable granules; fluctuant tumor mass

cm: Chronicity; infection

lb: Aspiration demonstrates straw-colored or bloody fluid

xr: Soft tissue swelling in prepatellar area; chronic cases often show radio-opaque bodies within bursa

pa: Synovitis within bursal sac

PROSTATITIS

et: Infection, usually nonspecific; may be secondary to gonorrhea; extension of inflammatory infectious diseases in other parts of body; heavy straining may be contributory

sm: Dysuria; burning, pain on urination; perineal pain; chills; backache

sg: Swelling, tenderness, enlargement of prostate; urethral discharge may be present; fever and weakness possible

cm: Chronicity

lb: Pyuria; leukocytosis

PUBIC SYMPHYSIS DISLOCATION

et: Direct blow; anteroposterior or lateral compression of pubis

sm: Pain over symphysis; inability to bear weight

sg: Local tenderness, swelling; sulcus at pubis may be palpated; pain elicited by gentle abduction of thigh

xr: True dislocation; or, may have vertical fracture through body of pubis near symphysis; or, wide separation of fragments may be present

PUBIS FRACTURE, INFERIOR RAMUS

et: Direct violence from front; lateral crushing injury
sm: Local pain; moderate disability
sg: Localized tenderness and swelling; pain elicited by abduction or hyperextension of thigh
xr: Fracture of inferior pubic ramus; little tendency for displacement

PUBIS FRACTURE, SUPERIOR RAMUS

et: Direct violence from front; lateral crushing injury
sm: Local pain; moderate disability
sg: Local tenderness and swelling; pain elicited by abduction or hyperextension of thigh
xr: Fracture of superior pubic ramus; little tendency for displacement

PULMONARY EMBOLISM

et: Venous thrombus especially from calf; trauma; postoperative complication; constricting bandage; impaction of dislodged clot ending in pulmonary artery
sm: Pain in chest; cough; hemoptysis, dyspnea; tachycardia; in severe cases: severe substernal pain; weakness; nausea; sweating; syncope
sg: Splinting of chest; shallow respirations; dullness to percussion; bronchial breath-sounds; rales; accentuation of pulmonic 2nd sound; pleuropericardial friction-rub; cyanosis; lowered blood pressure; dilatation of cervical veins; fever; acute distress with massive embolus; death
cm: Pulmonary edema; pleurisy with effusion; infection
lb: Leukocytosis; elevation of transaminase in serum; EKG: strain of right heart
xr: Small area of increased density, usually above diaphragm

PYELONEPHRITIS, ACUTE

et: Pyogenic bacteria; usually enteric bacilli, enterococcus, staphylococcus
sm: Chills; pain in lumbar region; frequency, oliguria, urgency, and dysuria; nausea, vomiting
sg: Rapid onset; costovertebral tenderness; fever
cm: Chronic pyelonephritis; hypertension
lb: Urine contains albumin, white blood cells with casts; leukocytosis; culture identification of organism
xr: Intravenous pyelography shows asymmetry of renal size, density of shadows

QUADRICEPS STRAIN

et: Excessive forcible use or stretching of quadriceps femoris; momentary incoordination, especially on fatigue; contraction suddenly arrested by outside force
sm: Stiffness, pain localized over front of thigh; disability
sg: Grade by degree of severity: muscle spasm, inflammation, swelling, followed by impaired function; ecchymosis may be remote from damaged tissue; possibly palpable defect
cm: Muscle hernia; formation of cyst, scar tissue

QUADRICEPS TENDON STRAIN

et: Indirect violence, as from stumbling, jumping, running
sm: Pain localized over tendon at its patellar attachment (upper pole); disability
sg: Grade by degree of severity: local tenderness, swelling; impaired knee extension; patella intact but sulcus may be palpable across torn tendon; hermarthrosis of knee
cm: Permanent weakness of knee extension

RADIOULNAR DISLOCATION, INFERIOR

et: Forcible hypersupination of wrist producing volar dislocation; forcible hyperpronation of wrist producing dorsal dislocation
sm: Pain on rotation of wrist; disability
sg: Increased prominence of ulnar head; limitation of rotation of wrist; swelling; tenderness over head of ulna; narrowing of wrist; clicking of wrist on rotation
xr: Alteration of distal radioulnar joint

RADIOULNAR FRACTURE

et: Fall onto outstretched hand; direct violence to forearm
sm: Pain; disability
sg: Deformity; swelling; tenderness; false motion; crepitus
cm: Volkmann's ischemic contracture; nonunion; angulation deformity; synosteosis
xr: Fracture of radial and ulnar shafts; variable type, depending upon force and mechanism

RADIUS DISLOCATION, HEAD

et: Indirect leverage force to forearm
sm: Pain; disability
sg: Elbow held in pronation and slight flexion; swelling, tenderness; pain elicited on passive flexion and supination of elbow; head of radius palpable in abnormal position
xr: Displaced head of radius

RADIUS FRACTURE, DISTAL EPIPHYSIS

at: Distal Radial Epiphysis Separation
et: Fall onto outstretched hand
sm: Pain; disability
sg: Silver fork deformity of distal radius; point tenderness; swelling; crepitus
cm: Alteration of epiphyseal growth
xr: Fracture of distal radial epiphysis; usually displaced dorsalward

RADIUS FRACTURE, HEAD-NECK

et: Blow directed upward, forcing radial head against distal end of humerus
sm: Pain at elbow; disability
sg: Local swelling, tenderness; defective rotation of forearm; deformity; crepitus on rotation; possibly hemarthrosis
xr: Fissure; marginal or comminuted fracture of radial head, neck; possibly displacement; may be associated with ulna fracture

RADIUS FRACTURE, SHAFT
et: Direct blow; fall onto outstretched hand with elbow in extension
sm: Local pain on pronation or supination; disability
sg: Spasm with deformity; tenderness; swelling
cm: Delayed union; malunion; persistent disability
xr: Usually greenstick type in children; oblique or comminuted with adults; may be associated with ulna fracture

RECTUS FEMORIS STRAIN
et: Change of stride while running; incoordination of muscles while running; fatigue; improper warmup prior to vigorous leg exercise
sm: Acute pain, anterior aspect of thigh; disability
sg: Grade by degree of severity: swelling; ecchymosis; tenderness localized over anterior aspect of thigh, midline; palpable defect possible; inability to extend affected thigh; pain elicited by active contraction of quadriceps group
cm: Recurrence; persistent disability

RHEUMATIC FEVER, ACUTE
et: Infection by beta hemolytic streptococcus (group A) followed by inflammation of connective tissue
sm: Insidious or abrupt onset usually in childhood; malaise; sweating; migrating pain in joints; prostration; palpitation; abdominal pain; epistaxis
sg: High fever; choreiform movements; tachycardia; cardiac enlargement with muffled sounds; polyarthritis; subcutaneous nodules
cm: Recurrent attacks; rheumatic heart disease with further complications
lb: Anemia; leukocytosis; proteinuria; C-reactive protein positive; titer of antistreptolysin high, decreasing with convalescence

RHINITIS, ACUTE
at: Common Cold
et: Virus infection
sm: Prodromal: dryness of nose, eyes, malaise, chills, headache. Later: nasal obstruction; sneezing; watery nasal discharge; lacrimation; postnasal drip; purulent discharge
cm: Secondary infection such as acute sinusitis, acute bronchitis

RIB FRACTURE
et: Direct or indirect trauma compressing chest; suddent violent muscular contraction
sm: Variable according to extent of injury; local pain; possibly dyspnea in multiple fracture as with collapse of chest wall
sg: Chest wall may be flattened, deformed; involved segment of chest displaced inward during inspiration (flail chest); crepitus; tenderness
cm: Damage to pleura, lung; pneumothorax; hemothorax; subcutaneous emphysema; shock
xr: Oblique or transverse fracture; frequently multiple, comminuted; overriding or minimal displacement; greenstick type in children

ROTATOR CUFF STRAIN, 1ST DEGREE
et: Fall onto outstretched arm; rapid, forced abduction of arm
sm: Minor pain; weakness
sg: Tenderness over upper end of humerus; weakness and loss of nor-

mal shoulder rhythm on either abduction or flexion
pa: Mild strain of rotator cuff muscles: supraspinatus, infraspinatus, and teres minor

ROTATOR CUFF STRAIN, 2ND DEGREE
et: Fall onto outstretched arm; rapid, forced abduction of arm
sm: Pain; moderate disability
sg: Weakness and loss of normal shoulder rhythm on either abduction or flexion; tenderness over upper end of humerus
pa: Incomplete or partial thickness tear of rotator cuff muscles: supraspinatus, infraspinatus, and teres minor; usually no direct communication between joint cavity and subacromial bursa

ROTATOR CUFF STRAIN, 3RD DEGREE
et: Fall onto outstretched arm; rapid, forced abduction of arm
sm: Pain; disability
sg: Weakness with inability to abduct shoulder actively through range of motion; tenderness over upper humerus; exquisite sensitivity at site of tear; rent may be palpable; crepitus; atrophy of affected muscles
xr: Athrography demonstrates defect in cuff
pa: Complete or full thickness tear of rotator cuff muscles: supraspinatus, infraspinatus, and teres minor; direct communication between joint cavity and subacromial bursa

SACROCOCCYGEAL DISLOCATION
et: Fall in sitting position
sm: Local pain; disability
sg: Local tenderness, swelling, ecchymosis; rectal examination indicates displacement, false motion, clicking
cm: Persistent disability
xr: Sacrococcygeal dislocation demonstrated

SACROILIAC DISLOCATION
et: Severe direct trauma from behind, or behind and laterally
sm: Local pain; inability to stand, sit, or turn over in bed
sg: Local tenderness, especially on compression of pelvis or manipulation of leg
cm: Persistent disability
xr: Dislocation of sacroiliac joint or associated vertical fracture through ilium or sacrum near joint; displacement rarely more than half inch

SACRUM FRACTURE
et: Direct violence from behind as from striking sacrum on edge of step from a fall
sm: Local pain; disability
sg: Local swelling, tenderness; false motion on rectal examination
xr: Fracture line roughly transverse at about level of lower end of sacroiliac joint; lower fragment may be displaced forward into pelvis; lateral view best

SARTORIUS STRAIN
et: Excessive forcible muscular action as in running or jumping
sm: Local pain over anterosuperior spine of ilium and along anterior aspect of thigh; disability

sg: Grade by degree of severity: swelling, tenderness near anterosuperior spine of ilium; pain elicited by passive external rotation of leg and by flexion or abduction of thigh
cm: Persistent disability; recurrence

SCAPULA FRACTURE

et: Direct blow; indirect trauma as in fall onto outstretched arm
sm: Local pain; disability
sg: Limited movement of arm; tenderness; swelling
xr: Body fracture: rarely displaced fragment; fracture lines linear or stellate, possibly extending to vertebral, axillary borders. Acromion process fracture: line possibly passing through base of acromion; slight displacement of fragment. Coracoid process fracture: fragment displacement. Spinous process fracture: slight fragment displacement. Glenoid fracture: chip or avulsion type; slight fragment displacement. Glenoid neck fracture: downward, inward displacement of plane at glenoid cavity

SCOLIOSIS

et: Primary: unknown, idiopathic. Secondary: underlying congenital or disease disorder. Sciatic: prolapsed intervertebral disc impinging upon lumbar or sacral nerve root. Compensatory: unequal leg length or fixed hip deformity
sm: Variable; occasional pain, aching; fatigue
sg: Lateral curvature of spine
cm: Deterioration of curve during rapid growth spurts; permanent deformity; neurological, cardiorespiratory dysfunction
xr: Determination of osseous involvement; may have secondary compensatory curves, rotation of vertebrae on vertical axis toward convexity of curve

SEBACEOUS CYST, INFECTED

at: Infected Wen
et: Bacterial infection of sebaceous cyst; scalp, face, back, ear, scrotum most common sites
sm: Local pain
sg: Inflamed discrete, movable subcutaneous mass; size of pea to walnut; purulent discharge mixed with cheesy, fatty material
cm: Abscess formation resembling furuncle

SHIN CONTUSION

at: Barked Shin
et: Direct blow to anterior tibial shaft
sm: Dull aching pain along crest of tibia; disability
sg: Local swelling, tenderness
cm: Secondary infection from accompanying abrasion, laceration; subperiosteal hematoma; periostitis

SINUS TARSI SYNDROME

et: Unknown; previous ankle sprain
sm: Pain persisting in sinus tarsi region long after ankle sprain; disability
sg: Tenderness and swelling localized over anterolateral aspect of foot below lateral malleolus; pain elicited by forced inversion of foot
cm: Persistent disability

SINUSITUS

et: Bacterial infection due to impaired drainage by engorged nasal mucosa in allergic or viral rhinitis; possibly changes in pressure during travel by air

sm: Headache, pain over affected sinus; malaise; anorexia; sometimes vertigo, anosmia, photophobia

sg: Tenderness over affected sinuses; nasal, postnasal discharge; fever; periorbital edema.

cm: Chronicity; bronchopneumonia; osteomyelitis of associated bones; brain abscess; meningitis

lb: Transillumination of frontal or maxillary sinuses poor or absent

xr: Cloudiness of affected sinuses; fluid level

*SKULL FRACTURE

et: Direct trauma to head

sm: Variable, depending on site and type of fracture; pain, headache, anosmia, visual and auditory disturbances, giddiness, nausea, vomiting, memory impairment; may be asymptomatic; moderate or severe concussion usually accompanies

sg: Altered state of consciousness; scalp edema or laceration; possibly blood in middle ear, cerebrospinal fluid rhinorrhea, otorrhea; nose bleed; contusion behind ear (Battle's sign); pupillary changes; possibly hemiparesis or hemiplegia, aphasia; pyramidal tract signs

cm: Cerebral laceration, contusion; extradural, subdural, or intracerebral hemorrhage; death

xr: Demonstrates type and extent of fracture: comminuted (fragmentation of bone); depressed (inward displacement of a part of the calvarium); diastatic (separation of cranial bones at a suture or marked separation of bone fragments); expressed (outward displacement of a part of the cranium); stellate (multiple radiating linear fracture); or, linear fracture

SMITH FRACTURE

at: Reversed Colles Fracture

et: Fall onto dorsum of hand

sm: Local pain; disability

sg: Deformity; swelling; possibly crepitus

cm: Malunion; Sudeck's syndrome; limitation of motion; carpal tunnel syndrome

xr: Fracture of distal radius with increase in volar angulation; possibly associated fracture of ulnar styloid process

SPERMATIC CORD TORSION

et: Parietal tunica revolving within scrotal tissue, usually in adolescence; abnormalities predisposing to torsion: abnormal motility of cord with incomplete attachment of epididymis to testicle; imperfect testicular descent; absent or long mesorchium; faulty development of gubernaculum

sm: Usually, sudden excruciating testicular pain, possibly referred along inguinal cord, lower abdomen; nausea, vomiting; may be asymptomatic at onset

sg: Swelling, tenderness of testis; scrotal edema, hyperemia; epididymis not palpated in usual posterior position

cm: Early detorsion necessary for prevention of gangrene, cord atrophy, loss of testis

SPINA BIFIDA OCCULTA

et: Congenital anomaly in spinous process and laminae of one or more vertebrae; herniation of spinal contents may not be present or noticeable; if of posterior type, skin may remain attached to membranes, nerve roots, or spinal cord; supporting ligaments underdeveloped; trauma aggravating factor

sm: May be asymptomatic; local low back pain, possibly radiating into buttocks

sg: Alterations of overlying skin: indentations, pigmentations, telangiectasis, or hairy patches; absent neurological manifestations; associated congenital deformities: clawfoot, clubfoot, scoliosis, kyphosis, lordosis, hip dislocation

cm: Spinal cord injury; infection

xr: Gap or defect in vertebral arch

*SPINAL CORD CONCUSSION

et: Direct blow to spine

sm: Clinical syndrome characterized by immediate and transient impairment of neural function; pain in back; numbness and weakness of extremities or trunk; interruption of normal bladder and bowel function with recovery

sg: Transient with recovery: paresis, paralysis, and abnormal tonus of extremities; loss in any or all sensory modalities to the level of lesion; usually areflexia; usually no pathologic reflexes

xr: Myelogram negative

pa: Transient neurophysiologic interruption

*SPINAL CORD CONTUSION

et: Direct blow to spine with structural alteration of spinal cord characterized by extravasation of blood cells and tissue necrosis with edema

sm: Weakness or paralysis of extremities and trunk; numbness of extremities and trunk to level of lesion; bladder and bowel dysfunction

sg: Partial or permanent impairment of neural function; paresis, paralysis of extremities and trunk; varying degrees of sensory modality loss consistent with extent and level of lesion; hyperreflexia with pyramidal tract signs

lb: Cerebrospinal fluid may show blood cells or elevated protein; may show partial block on jugular vein compression test

xr: May show associated fracture; myelogram may show partial or complete block if edema is present

SPINAL CORD HEMATOMYELIA

at: Intramedullary Spinal Hemorrhage

et: Trauma; spontaneous; congential; central hemorrhage secondary to cyst formation or infarction in center of cord

sm: Acute onset; numbness, tingling of fingers and hands, paralysis of hands, arms, and subsequently legs, with loss of pain sense

sg: Alteration of superficial pain and temperature sense; spastic weakness first in upper extremities, then in lower extremities; associated sensory loss; disturbance of bladder and bowel control; usually flaccid paraplegia early, spastic late

cm: In acute stage, possible ascending paralysis with respiratory failure; if chronic, marked weakness usually in both upper extremities with atrophy and contractures, possible skin ulcerations

xr: Possible associated fracture-dislocation of spine in acute trauma; myelogram may demonstrate widening of canal and filling defect particularly in cervical area

SPINAL CORD SYNDROME, ACUTE, ANTERIOR CERVICAL

et: Usually associated with flexion injury of cervical spine with or without fracture or fracture-dislocation, frequently with "tear drop" fracture, rarely with herniated cervical disc

sm: Immediate complete paralysis of trunk and all extremities with numbness below the site of the lesion; bladder and bowel dysfunction

sg: Complete flaccid paralysis of all muscles below lesion; areflexia; loss of pain and temperature senses to level of lesion but preservation of motion, position, and vibration sensation

cm: Possibly permanent tetraplegia

lb: No block on Queckenstedt test; cerebrospinal fluid may contain red blood cells; protein may be elevated

xr: May show vertebral body injury if present

*SPINAL CORD SYNDROME, ACUTE, CENTRAL CERVICAL

at: Schneider's Syndrome

et: Forcible hyperextension of cervical spine; squeeze of cervical cord between osteophyte anteriorly in spinal canal and the wrinkled ligamentum flavum; or, vascular insufficiency by compression of vertebral arteries; complete recovery possible

sm: Disproportionately greater weakness in upper extremities than lower; urinary retention; varying degrees of sensory loss

sg: Immediate complete paralysis of fingers, forearms and arms with paresis in the proximal muscles of the lower extremities; movement in feet possible; if due to vascular insufficiency, nerve root pain and no loss of sensation at site of lesion; complete sensory loss possible with spinal cord squeeze

cm: Possible permanent damage with paralysis of upper extremities and loss of bladder and bowel control

lb: No block on Queckenstedt test; possibly protein elevation in cerebrospinal fluid

xr: Osteoarthritic spurs on posterior portion of body of cervical vertebrae; or, may find fracture-dislocation or fracture of vertebral body

pa: Central hemorrhagic destruction or central edematomyelia of cervical spinal cord

SPINAL HEMORRHAGE, EXTRADURAL

at: Epidural Spinal Hemorrhage

et: Trauma; usually associated with penetrating wound or a greenstick fracture of a rheumatoid spondylitic cervical spine; spontaneous onset with anticoagulants; usually of venous origin unless associated with rheumatoid spondylitis fracture

sm: Pain in neck, usually progressive with rather severe pain radiating downward into the scapular and dorsal spinal areas; most severe cases show partial or complete paralysis of extremities on the basis of spinal cord compression; numbness from site of lesion downward; bladder and bowel impairment

sg: Stiff neck and limitation of motion; severe pain on local percussion;

gradual paresis, partial or complete; early areflexic involvement; subsequent bilateral pyramidal tract signs

cm: Permanent paralysis, either tetraplegia or paraplegia, with bladder and bowel dysfunction; if ascending, respiratory paralysis and death

lb: May have increased protein in cerebrospinal fluid or a block on the Queckenstedt test

xr: May demonstrate spinal fracture; occasionally a penetrating wound will be source of difficulty with foreign body noted on x-ray

SPINAL HEMORRHAGE, SUBDURAL

et: Rare; associated with trauma to spine with or without fracture or penetrating wound; may be due to rupture of arteriovenous malformation

sm: Pain in back; ascending weakness of arms and legs; gradually increased bladder impairment

sg: Paresis in lower extremities progressing to paralysis extending to upper extremities if site of lesion is cervical; dysfunction of bladder and bowel; may show Brown-Sequard pattern; increased reflexes early, later becoming flaccid; pyramidal tract signs

cm: Permanent paralysis, bladder dysfunction

lb: Lumbar puncture shows partial or complete block of cerebrospinal fluid

SPINE DISLOCATION, ATLANTOAXIAL

at: Atlantoaxial Subluxation

et: Congenital weakness of ligaments; congenital absence of odontoid process; head trauma causing disruption of ligaments; inflammatory reaction producing relaxation of ligaments

sm: Pain in neck; difficulty of rotating head into normal plane

sg: Cervical muscle spasm; headache, suboccipital or vertex; tendency to maintain head in slightly forward position or tilted to one side

cm: Excessive subluxation may result in high cervical cord compression, vertebral artery compression, hypoxia, and death

xr: Lateral view may show absence of odontoid process or dislocation of atlas on axis, anteriorly most frequently; open mouth view shows fracture of odontoid base. CAUTION: flexion and extension views with or without laminography demonstrate degree of subluxation

SPINE DISLOCATION, CERVICAL ARTICULAR PROCESS

at: Overriding Facets; Locked Facets; Jumped-process Complex

et: Usually a severe twisting or wrench type of neck injury; may also be lateral blow to head or cervical spine: diving in shallow water; infection with relaxation of joints in childhood

sm: Pinched nerve syndrome if spontaneous reduction; usually unilateral with pain in neck with and without movement; may have pain and/or numbness radiating into arm, forearm, and fingers; if bilateral, may result in both spinal cord and nerve root impairment with complete paralysis or weakness with numbness to level of lesion; inability to urinate or defecate; respiratory difficulty

sg: If unilateral: radicular pain with downward thrust of head; paresis, numbness, and possibly areflexia; tilt of head to opposite side. If bilateral: may have various stages from asymptomatic to complete areflexic tetraplegia (with bladder and bowel dysfunction)

cm: Bilateral lesions may result in partial or complete permanent paralysis

lb: EMG after three weeks may show degree of root impairment; protein elevated in cerebrospinal fluid; possible block on jugular vein compression test

xr: Demonstrates complete dislocation of one or both articular facets, usually with overriding of the inferior articular process of the vertebra above into a position anterior to the superior articular process of the vertebra below; laminograms may reveal degree of dislocation and possibly presence of fracture line through facets

*SPINE FRACTURE, COMPRESSION

at: Wedge Vertebral Fracture
et: Forcible flexion spinal injury; blow on head as in diving in shallow water; fall from height onto feet
sm: Local variable pain; with nerve root compression: numbness, radicular pain in chest and extremities, unilaterally or bilaterally; with spinal cord compression: weakness or paralysis, perhaps numbness in trunk and extremities, bladder and bowel dysfunction
sg: Percussion elicits radicular pain or local pain over spine, accentuated on any movement; may have radicular hypesthesia or muscular weakness; in extreme cases, tetraplegia, areflexia, bladder dysfunction, and partial to complete sensory impairment, pathological reflexes
cm: Possible subsequent neurological deficit if spine is unstable
lb: May show block on Queckenstedt test; protein may be elevated in cerebrospinal fluid
xr: Break in continuity of vertebra with narrowing of its vertical height, particularly at the most anterior portion of the vertebral body

SPINE FRACTURE, HANGMAN'S

at: Cervical Spine Axial Arch Avulsion Fracture
et: Sudden deceleration in hyperextension of cervical spine
sm: Local pain; restriction of any movement of neck
sg: Tenderness; pain elicited by movement of neck; usually associated with no neurological deficit other than transient radicular hypesthesia over face; hemihypesthesia (rare)
cm: Continued or progressive dislocation with possible high cervical cord compression and death
xr: Lateral view shows bilateral axial arch avulsion with possible anterior dislocation of C2 on C3 vertebral body

SPINE FRACTURE, SPINOUS PROCESS

et: Direct blow to spine; sudden forcible twisting or wrenching movement
sm: Pain localized over involved spinous process
sg: Local tenderness on percussion over involved spinous process
xr: Lateral view shows fracture of spinous process

*SPINE FRACTURE, 'TEARDROP'

at: Explosive Cervical Fracture
et: Forcible flexion of cervical spine as in diving into shallow water
sm: If uncomplicated, pain in neck only; if subluxation present, nerve root compression may produce numbness, weakness, and pain in muscles of upper extremity; if dislocation present, immediate tetraplegia may occur
sg: Varying degree of severity: If slight, none. If moderate, nerve root compression unilaterally or bilaterally with radicular discomfort,

weakness or numbness in upper extremities. If severe, anterior cord compression by posterior margin of split vertebra protruding posteriorly into spinal canal against cord producing acute anterior cervical spinal cord syndrome

cm: Possibly complete tetraplegia; late collapse of vertebral body with laying down of bone in spinal canal causing chronic compression syndrome

lb: Negative to moderate elevated protein in cerebrospinal fluid

xr: Anterior inferior portion of vertebra slipping away from vertebral body above it; protrustion of the posteroinferior margin of the involved vertebral body into spinal canal; myelogram in chronic phase shows impingement on spinal canal and cervical spinal cord

SPINE FRACTURE, TRANSVERSE PROCESS

et: Direct blow to spine; sudden forcible twisting or wrenching movement

sm: Pain localized over site of fracture, especially on movement

sg: Local tenderness over site of fracture

cm: Renal injury frequently associated

xr: Anteroposterior view demonstrates fracture of transverse process

SPINE FRACTURE-DISLOCATION

at: Spine Subluxation

et: Cervical: forcible flexion, lateral or rotary twisting of head and neck; blow to head as in diving. Thoracic: forcible flexion as in wrestling. Lumbar: fall from height, landing on buttocks

sm: Local pain without neurological deficit if simple spine lesion; radicular pain, numbness, and weakness in upper extremity if associated with root involvement; often associated with spinal cord injury with symptoms appropriate to level of lesion

sg: Variable from none to complete neurologic deficit according to level and degree of nerve injury; tenderness on percussion if limited to simple spine lesion

cm: Permanent tetraplegia or paraplegia

lb: Lumbar puncture may show block on Queckenstedt test, elevated red or white blood cell count, elevated protein

xr: Fracture-dislocation of one vertebral body on another, perhaps associated with other bony disruption; far more bony damage present than viewed on film

SPLEEN CONTUSION

et: Trauma to left thorax, abdomen, especially in contact sports; enlarged spleen from disease such as infectious mononucleosis contributory

sm: Upper abdominal pain, possibly referred to left shoulder; nausea, vomiting; dizziness, syncope

sg: Pallor; rigidity in left hypochondrium; tachycardia; shock

cm: Ruptured spleen

lb: Anemia; leukocytosis

SPLEEN RUPTURE

et: Trauma to left thorax, abdomen, especially in contact sports; enlarged spleen from disease such as infectious mononucleosis contributory

sm: Upper abdominal pain, usually referred to the left shoulder; nausea; weakness; syncope sg: Pallor; rigidity of abdominal muscles; tachycardia; falling blood pressure; shock

cm: Irreversible shock, death if blood not promptly replaced and spleen surgically removed

lb: Falling hemoglobin and hematocrit; abdominal paracentesis may yield blood

xr: May demonstrate enlarged spleen; fluid level in pelvis in erect position; increased density in left upper quadrant in Trendelenburg position

SPONDYLITIS, RHEUMATOID

at: Ankylosing Spondylitis; Strumpell-Marie Disease; Atrophic Spinal Arthritis

et: Unknown; usually occurs in males between ages 20-35

sm: Pain begins in lower back with increasing stiffness; later, pain migrates upwards and radiates downward to one or both lower limbs

sg: Variable and progressive: tenderness; gradual limitation of all movements in area of spine; gradual loss of chest expansion; head fixed in forward displacement (later stage)

cm: Permanent stiffness; gross flexion deformity of spine; severe disability

xr: Early: loss of clear joint outline in both sacroiliac joints, best seen with 35° oblique view. Later: sacroiliac joints completely obliterated and, if disease progresses, intervertebral joints in upper spine undergo bony ankylosis; calcified anterior and lateral ligaments; rarefaction of vertebral bodies

pa: Chronic ascending inflammation of joints of spinal column beginning with sacroiliac

SPONDYLOLISTHESIS, LUMBAR

et: Unknown; spondylolysis or congenital malformation of articular processes predisposing

sm: May be asymptomatic; chronic backache, with or without sciatica, aggravated on standing; may be referred to buttocks

sg: Visible or palpable step above sacral crest; exaggerated lumbar lordosis; impairment of straight-leg raising

cm: Possible progressive displacement; sciatica; irritation of one of issuing nerves; persistent disabling low back pain

xr: Displacement of a lumbar vertebral body upon segment below it, usually forward; oblique views show neural arch defect which allows separation of vertebra's two halves, the body going forward, leaving laminae and inferior articular processes behind

SPONDYLOLYSIS, LUMBAR

et: Unknown; congenital or acquired defect in neural arch of lumbar vertebra, usually L5

sm: Variable; asymptomatic to deep chronic low back pain; symptoms increased on weight bearing

sg: Variable degree of restriction of spinal movements

cm: Spondylolisthesis if defect stretches or gives; traumatic arthritis; disability

xr: Oblique film demonstrates defect in neural arch

pa: Loss of bony continuity between superior and inferior articular processes; deficiency bridged by fibrous tissue

*SPONDYLOSIS, CERVICAL

at: Cervical Traumatic Arthritis
et: Reactive changes in cervical vertebral bodies about the interspace associated with chronic discopathy from trauma incident or repeated episodes of trauma
sm: Pain in neck, headache or radicular discomfort on movement; weakness and numbness in extremities and trunk
sg: May show unsteady gait; neck pain elicited on movement, especially toward side of lesion; radicular hypesthesia and paresis of upper extremities; impaired biceps or triceps reflexes; with cord compression, paresis to paralysis of upper or lower extremities, increased tonus in extremities, patellar and ankle clonus, hyperreflexia, pyramidal tract signs, hypalgesia to level of lesion
cm: Spinal cord damage
lb: May have partial block on jugular vein compression test; elevated protein
xr: Lateral and oblique views show narrowing of intervertebral space with bony overgrowth, bony spurs on anterior and posterior margins of vertebrae; vertebral bodies may be subluxated; myelogram positive for root impingement or midline bony bars

*SPONDYLOSIS, LUMBAR

at: Lumbar Traumatic Arthritis
et: Reactive changes in vertebral lumbar bodies about the interspace associated with chronic discopathy from trauma incident or repeated minor episodes of trauma
sm: Back or radicular pain; may have weakness, bladder and bowel dysfunction
sg: Hypalgesia, paresis in lower extremities; bladder or bowel incontinence; hyporeflexia to areflexia
cm: Chronicity
lb: May have partial block on jugular vein compression test; elevated protein
xr: Lateral and oblique views show narrowing of intervertebral space with bony overgrowth, bony spurs on anterior and posterior margins of vertebrae; vertebral bodies may be subluxated; myelogram positive for root impingement or midline bony bars

SPRAIN, 1ST DEGREE

at: Mild Sprain
et: Direct or indirect trauma to joint
sm: Pain; mild disability
sg: Mild point tenderness; no abnormal motion; little or no swelling; minimal hemorrhage; minimal functional loss
cm: Tendency to recurrence, aggravation
pa: Minor tearing of ligament fibers

SPRAIN, 2ND DEGREE

at: Moderate Sprain
et: Direct or indirect trauma to joint
sm: Pain; moderate disability
sg: Point tenderness; moderate loss of function; slight to moderate abnormal motion; swelling; localized hemorrhage
cm: Tendency to recurrence, aggravation; persistent instability; traumatic arthritis
pa: Partial tear of ligament

SPRAIN, 3RD DEGREE

at: Severe Sprain
et: Severe direct or indirect trauma to joint
sm: Pain; disability
sg: Loss of function; marked abnormal motion; possible deformity; tenderness; swelling; hemorrhage
cm: Persistent instability; traumatic arthritis
xr: Stress film demonstrates abnormal motion
pa: Complete tear of ligament

STERNOCLAVICULAR SPRAIN, 1ST DEGREE

et: Blow to lateral aspect of shoulder; shoulder suddenly forced forward
sm: Minimal pain, disability
sg: No laxity of joint; no deformity; point tenderness
pa: Minor tearing of sternoclavicular and costoclavicular ligament fibers

STERNOCLAVICULAR SPRAIN, 2ND DEGREE

at: Sternoclavicular Subluxation
et: Blow to lateral aspect of shoulder; shoulder suddenly forced forward
sm: Local pain; disability
sg: Swelling; moderate deformity; point tenderness
pa: Complete rupture of sternoclavicular ligament and partial tear of costoclavicular ligament

STERNOCLAVICULAR SPRAIN, 3RD DEGREE

at: Sternoclavicular Dislocation
et: Severe blow to lateral aspect of shoulder; shoulder suddenly forced forward
sm: Local pain; disability
sg: Marked deformity with displacement anteriorly or retrosternally; point tenderness; swelling; respiratory distress
cm: Traumatic arthritis; recurrence; retrosternal displacement may cause great vessel damage, death
xr: Oblique views demonstrate displacement; tomography and laminography may be necessary
pa: Complete rupture of sternoclavicular and costoclavicular ligaments

STERNUM FRACTURE

et: Direct or indirect trauma; may be associated with compression fracture of spine
sm: Local pain
sg: Deformity; ecchymosis; tenderness; possibly palpable offset
xr: Fracture line usually at junction of manubrium and sternal body; possible displacement

STING, INSECT

et: Venom transmitted by bee, wasp, hornet, ant through punctate wound
sm: Sharp pain; intense pruritus; nausea; abdominal cramps; malaise
sg: Rapid swelling; wheal; erythema; sometimes urticaria; stinger may be present in wound
cm: Sensitization; anaphylaxis; death

STITCH IN SIDE

at: Runner's Ache; Catch in Side
et: Unknown; thought to be from stretching of large intestine by gas pockets accumulated by jostling in running, constipation, local anoxia, or spasm of diaphragm
sm: Sharp pain in side, usually right side while running; somewhat disabling; relief after cessation of activity
sg: Obvious distress

STRAIN, 1ST DEGREE

at: Mild Strain; Slightly Pulled Muscle
et: Trauma to portion of musculotendinous unit from excessive forcible use or stretch
sm: Local pain, aggravated by movement or tension of muscle; minor disability
sg: Mild spasm, swelling, ecchymosis; local tenderness; minor loss of function and strength
cm: Tendency to recurrence, aggravation; tendinitis; periostitis at attachment
pa: No appreciable hemorrhage, being confined to low grade inflammation and some disruption of muscle-tendon tissue

STRAIN, 2ND DEGREE

at: Moderate Strain; Moderately Pulled Muscle
et: Trauma to portion of musculotendinous unit from violent contraction or excessive forcible stretch, often associated with failure in synergistic action
sm: Local pain, aggravated by movement or tension of muscle; moderate disability
sg: Moderate spasm, swelling, ecchymosis; local tenderness; impaired muscle function
cm: Tendency to recurrence, aggravation
pa: Stretching and tearing of fibers without complete disruption

STRAIN, 3RD DEGREE

at: Severe Strain; Severely Pulled Muscle
et: Trauma to portion of musculotendinous unit from violent contraction or excessive forcible stretch, often associated with failure in synergistic action
sm: Severe pain; disability
sg: Severe spasm; swelling, ecchymosis; hematoma; tenderness, loss of muscle function; defect usually palpable
cm: Prolonged disability
xr: May see avulsion fracture at tendinous attachment, soft tissue swelling
pa: Muscle or tendon ruptured separating muscle from muscle, muscle from tendon, or avulsion of tendon from bone

STY, EXTERNAL

at: External Hordeolum
et: Infection of minute gland in eyelid, usually by staphylococcus; frequently associated with acne vulgaris of face
sm: Lacrimation; photophobia; sensation of presence of foreign body in eye; pain

sg: Hyperemic area on margin of lid spreading, becoming tender area of induration; small boil-like lesion with yellow spot in center
cm: Extension of infection, possibly due to direct trauma

SUBACROMIAL BURSITIS
at: Scapulohumeral Bursitis; Subdeltoid Bursitis
et: Attrition; acute or chronic trauma; possibly inflammation secondary to necrosis
sm: Severe pain in shoulder region radiating to neck, arm, finger tips
sg: Marked tenderness over greater tuberosity; local swelling and distention; pain aggravated by abduction and/or rotation of arm; limitation of motion
cm: Calcified bursitis; supraspinatus tendinitis with or without calcification
lb: Leukocytosis
xr: May have opaque rounded shadow of calcium deposit overlying head of humerus, localized atrophy of adjacent bone
pa: Inflammation of bursa with partial rupture of tendon of small rotator muscles

SUBTALAR-TALONAVICULAR DISLOCATION
et: Fall from height; excessive forcible torsion of foot
sm: Severe pain; complete disability
sg: Marked swelling; foot fixed in abnormal position on leg; malleoli intact; if foot displaced backward, head of talus palpable in front of ankle and forefoot shortened; if foot displaced forward, a prominence beneath achilles tendon is seen and heel shortened; if lateral, displacement readily seen
cm: Impaired circulation to foot; traumatic arthritis
xr: Talus out of subtalar and talonavicular joints but remaining in ankle mortise; foot displaced forward, inward, backward or outward on foot

SUPERIOR TIBIOFIBULAR DISLOCATION
at: Upper End Fibula Dislocation
et: Direct violence; severe leverage forces
sm: Pain; disability
sg: Obvious deformity of head of fibula; tenderness
cm: Compression of peroneal nerve; prolonged disabliity
xr: Dislocation may be backward, forward, outward, or upward

TALUS DISLOCATION
at: Astragalus Dislocation
et: Fall from height onto foot
sm: Severe pain; complete disability
sg: Obvious deformity; extensive swelling; malleoli lowered on calcaneous; foot may be displaced backward or forward on leg
cm: Supervening infection; traumatic arthritis; aseptic necrosis of talus
xr: Total dislocation of talus forward and outward, or inward, or backward

TALUS FRACTURE, BODY
at: Astragalus Fracture
et: Fall from height onto feet
sm: Pain on movement; inability to bear weight

sg: Swelling and tenderness in front of and behind malleoli; no puffiness of heel; no apparent deformity

cm: Nonunion; aseptic necrosis of proximal fragment; traumatic arthritis

xr: Fracture through body of talus; may be displaced or nondisplaced; telescoping; disorganization of articular surfaces

TALUS FRACTURE, DOME, OSTEOCHONDRAL, SUPEROLATERAL MARGIN

at: Flake Fracture of Talus Dome; Osteochondritis Dissecans of Talus Dome

et: Excessive forcible eversion-dorsiflexion of foot; snubbing type of fracture; cartilage of superolateral surface of talus is peeled off subchondral bone taking a fragment of bone with it

sm: Pain persisting despite treatment, aggravated by activity, subsiding with rest; catching in ankle

sg: Tenderness over anterolateral confluence of tibia, fibula, and talus; crepitus

cm: Irreversible chronic arthritic changes in joint cartilage and in capsular structure

xr: Crater appearing in articular surface, occupied by a line of opacity, surrounded by an area of radiolucency

TALUS FRACTURE, DOME, OSTEOCHONDRAL, SUPEROMEDIAL MARGIN

at: Flake Fracture of Talus Dome; Osteochondritis Dissecans of Talus Dome

et: Excessive forcible inversion-plantarflexion of foot as in landing on toes with foot inverted

sm: Pain persisting despite treatment, aggravated by activity, subsiding with rest; catching in ankle

sg: Tenderness over superomedial side of foot; crepitus

cm: Irreversible chronic arthritic changes in joint cartilage and in capsular structure

xr: Dislodged talar cartilage with some subchondral bone on posterior end of superomedial surface of talus; crater in articular surface, occupied by a line of opacity, surrounded by an area of radiolucency

TALUS FRACTURE, HEAD

et: Excessive forcible dorsiflexion of foot

sm: Pain; disability

sg: Local tenderness over dorsum of foot at talonavicular joint; swelling

cm: Persistent disability; traumatic arthritis

xr: Relatively large fragment of bone broken off talar head

TALUS FRACTURE, HEAD, AVULSION

et: Excessive forcible plantarflexion of foot

sm: Pain localized just proximal to talonavicular joint over dorsum of foot; disability

sg: Local tenderness and swelling; avulsed fragment may be palpable; pain elicited by active plantarflexion

cm: Persistent disability

xr: Avulsion fracture of superior margin of talus head; slight displacement dorsally and proximally

TALUS FRACTURE, NECK

et: Fall onto foot; talus crushed between tibia and calcaneus with shearing force
sm: Pain; disability
sg: Forefoot displaced slightly upward and inward on heel; marked swelling and tenderness at front of ankle; deep palpation of sharp proximal edge of distal fragment; with posterior displacement of body, marked swelling beneath achilles tendon
cm: Traumatic arthritis; chronic disability; aseptic necrosis of talar body
xr: Transverse fracture of talar neck with upward and inward displacement of distal or head fragment; or, vertical fracture through neck posteriorly, with posterior portion displaced backward, tilting so fracture surface points downward against calcaneus

TALUS FRACTURE, POSTERIOR PROCESS

et: Violent force transmitted upward through heel; excessive plantarflexion of foot
sm: Pain in region posterior to malleoli; disability
sg: Slight swelling and tenderness posterior to malleoli; pain elicited by flexing or extending ankle
cm: Nonunion
xr: Loose fragment of posterior process displaced backward and upward

TALUS FRACTURE, POSTERIOR PROCESS AVULSION

et: Excessive forcible dorsiflexion of foot
sm: Pain deep behind achilles tendon posteriorly in midline; disability
sg: Local tenderness; pain elicited by active dorsiflexion of foot
xr: Avulsed fragment of posterior portion of talus

TARSAL TUNNEL SYNDROME

et: Unknown; thin band of fibrous tissue extending from flexor retinaculum compressing tibial nerve as it passes beneath
sm: Burning paresthesia of foot, mostly at night, relieved by hanging leg out of bed or walking
sg: Sensory loss from base of big toe to about medial border of sole and in a wide band along lateral edge; dorsum not affected; small nodular swelling behind medial malleolus just above posterior margin of flexor retinaculum
cm: Persistent disability
lb: Nerve conduction-time studies abnormal for posterior tibial nerve

TARSAL NAVICULAR FRACTURE

at: Tarsal Scaphoid Fracture
et: Force transmitted upward from forefoot through cuneiform bones, compressing navicular between these bones and head of talus; fall onto ball of foot; excessive forcible dorsiflexion or torsion of foot
sm: Pain in region over navicular; inability to bear weight
sg: Medial fragment may be palpable on anterior border of foot; foot tends to be held in eversion; pain elicited by inversion or dorsiflexion of foot
cm: Nonunion; traumatic arthritis; persistent stiffness, pain
xr: Fracture line tends to be vertical across body of navicular, or tuberosity may be broken off, or bone may be comminuted; medial

fragment tends to be displaced inward or upward; navicular may instead be crushed upward from below and compressed; laminography may be extremely helpful

TARSAL NAVICULAR FRACTURE, AVULSION

et: Excessive forcible plantarflexion of foot
sm: Pain localized over dorsum of foot near talonavicular joint
sg: Local tenderness and swelling; pain elicited by plantarflexion of foot
cm: Persistent disability
xr: Avulsion fracture of superior lip of tarsal navicular with slight displacement

TARSAL NAVICULAR FRACTURE, OSTEOCHONDRAL

et: Fall from height
sm: Pain localized to dorsum of foot at talonavicular joint
sg: Local tenderness and swelling; pain elicited by forced motions of foot
cm: Traumatic arthritis; persistent disability
xr: Small fragment involving superior margin of posterior surface of tarsal navicular with a translucent area between it and parent bone, giving crater-like appearance at cartilage surface

TARSOMETATARSAL DISLOCATION

et: Fall onto ball of foot; direct crushing injury; excessive forcible torsion of foot
sm: Pain; disability
sg: Marked swelling of entire forefoot; obvious deformity; dorsal dislocation shows marked prominence on dorsum of foot where thick base of metatarsal dislocates, extensor tendons drawn tightly over prominence; lateral dislocation usually visible as well as palpable; pain elicited on abduction and adduction of foot
cm: Persistent stiffness, pain; traumatic arthritis
xr: Entire group of metatarsals may be dislocated upon tarsal bones, displacement being lateral, upward, or downward; or, a single metatarsal is dislocated and displaced upward; or, two or more may be dislocated upward, downward, or laterally; 1st and 5th most frequently affected

TEMPOROMANDIBULAR DISLOCATION

at: Dislocated Jaw
et: Sudden violent trauma; sudden exaggerated opening of jaw
sm: Severe local pain; locking of jaw
sg: Obvious deformity; mouth fixed in open position; defect palpable; displacement of condyles anterior to normal position; or, displacement of mandible toward opposite side

TENDINITIS

et: Degenerative changes secondary to repeated minor trauma and circulatory disturbance; attrition; associated with various types of arthritis; infection
sm: Pain; limited motion of affected part; fatigue
sg: Erythema; swelling; crepitus; impaired function
cm: Adhesions; calcific deposits

105

TENOSYNOVITIS

et: Unknown; possible causative factors: direct blow or repeated trauma; unaccustomed forcible use of tendon's muscle
sm: Pain; limited motion of affected part
sg: Tenderness over tendon; swelling; crepitus
cm: Constrictive adhesions
pa: Inflammation between tendon and surrounding tissues with consequent loss of smooth gliding motion

TENOSYNOVITIS, STENOSING

at: Trigger Finger; deQuervain's Disease
et: Constriction of tendon in its sheath by its retaining fibrous ligament, usually due to repetitive trauma
sm: Painful snapping and locking on function
sg: Tenderness; local palpable nodule
pa: Three sites: 1st dorsal compartment of wrist involving tendons of abductor pollicis longus and extensor pollicis brevis; sheaths of flexor sublimus and profundus tendons of two middle fingers in palm; sheath of flexor pollicus longus at metacarpophalangeal joint

TESTIS INJURY

et: Contusion as from kick, direct blow, or fall on hard object
sm: Severe pain; nausea, vomiting
sg: Contusion; laceration; swelling; ecchymosis; tenderness; extravasation of blood
cm: Necrosis; hematoma; orchitis; gangrene; atrophy; sterility; atrophy of epididymis

TETANUS

at: Lockjaw
et: Exotoxin of clostridium tetani, introduced through open wound, usually puncture wound or wounds with devitalized tissue; incubation period three days to four weeks
sm: Restlessness; difficulty in swallowing; muscle cramps and spasms; severe pain
sg: Persistent spasm of muscles near site of wound; increase of muscle tone of various groups; difficulty in swallowing; later, stiffness, rigidity of neck, trunk, and extremities; fever
cm: Often ends in death; asphyxia during spasm; pneumonia; urinary retention; compression fracture of vertebrae
lb: Culture of little value

THROMBOPHLEBITIS

et: Unknown; veins of calf most common site. Possible causative factors: intimal damage of vein, venous stasis, changes in coagulating properties of blood. Predisposing: surgical operations, trauma, shock, burns, prolonged bed rest
sm: May be asymptomatic; pain, discomfort in leg; variable disability
sg: Variable with site; swelling; tenderness; erythema; fever; local cyanosis; may have positive Homan's sign
cm: Postphlebitic syndrome; postsurgical recurrences; pulmonary embolism
lb: Blood pressure cuff elicits severe pain between 80-120 mm Hg; sedimentation rate may be elevated

TIBIA FRACTURE, LATERAL CONDYLE

at: Tibia Fracture, Lateral Plateau
et: Force applied to lateral side of extended knee; fall onto feet with leg being bowed inward; sharp edge of lateral femoral condyle rotates slightly medially and drives into central portion of lateral tibial plateau
sm: Pain; major disability
sg: Local tenderness, swelling; hemarthrosis; valgus deformity possible; abduction instability of knee possible
cm: Malunion; traumatic arthritis; instability
xr: Displacement of edge of tibial plateau laterally; depression of central portion of plateau

TIBIA FRACTURE, LATERAL CONDYLE AVULSION

et: Excessive forcible adduction of leg
sm: Pain; disability
sg: Swelling, hemarthrosis; tenderness over lateral tibial condyle; varus deformity possible; abnormal varus mobility of leg inward
cm: Persistent instability
xr: Avulsion of fragment of lateral tibial condyle, displaced upward; oblique views best

TIBIA FRACTURE, MEDIAL CONDYLE

et: Direct or indirect violence; fall onto feet with leg being bowed outward; excessive forcible adduction of leg
sm: Pain; disability
sg: Swelling, hemarthrosis; variable varus deformity; tenderness; possible broadening of region below knee; abnormal varus mobility of leg
cm: Malunion; traumatic arthritis
lb: Aspiration shows blood containing fat particles
xr: Small triangular section of medial condyle split off and displaced downward and impacted; fragment may be larger, split may be vertical and inner edge displaced medially; margin of medial condyle may be crushed downward; oblique views or laminograms helpful

TIBIA FRACTURE, MEDIAL CONDYLE AVULSION

et: Excessive forcible abduction of leg
sm: Pain; disability
sg: Swelling; hemarthrosis; tenderness; possible valgus deformity; abnormal valgus mobility of leg
cm: Persistent instability
xr: Avulsion of fragment of medial tibial condyle pulled upward; oblique views helpful

TIBIA FRACTURE, POSTERIOR RIM AVULSION

et: Forcible hyperextension; blow to front of fixed leg with knee in flexion
sm: Pain in back of knee; disability
sg: Swelling; hemarthrosis; tibia displaced posteriorly; ecchymosis
cm: Instability
xr: Avulsion of posterior rim of tibia by posterior cruciate ligament

TIBIA FRACTURE, SHAFT

et: Direct or indirect violence; fall onto feet from height; excessive forcible torsion as with foot or thigh fixed while other end is twisted

sm: Pain; inability to bear weight

sg: Possible shortening of leg; possible deformity: angulation of leg or rotation of foot; variable amount of swelling and tenderness; pain elicited by compression or rotating foot with knee immobilized or by pushing foot upward

cm: Malunion; nonunion; delayed union; tibiofibular synosteosis; impaired circulation and nerve supply to foot

xr: Transverse, oblique, spiral, comminuted, anterior, posterior, medial or lateral displacement, overriding, segmental, butterfly fragment, greenstick, rotation fractures; distal end of proximal fragment tends to occupy position anterior and lateral to proximal end of distal fragment which tends to be rotated outward

TIBIA FRACTURE, SHAFT, FATIGUE

at: Tibia March Fracture; Tibia Stress Fracture

et: Excessive repetitive activity, especially among adolescents

sm: Local pain while running, jumping, increasing gradually

sg: Small tender hard lump about middle of tibial crest or along posteromedial margin of tibia; erythema

xr: Initially negative; after 2-3 weeks, horizontal fissure with adjacent hyperostosis; linear rarefaction running into bone with some thickening of overlying periosteum

TIBIA FRACTURE, SPINE

at: Tibia Spine Fracture Avulsion

et: Fracture of lateral tubercle, produced by sharp inner margin of lateral femoral condyle as leg is externally rotated and driven backward and flexed upon femur; avulsion of tibial spine at anterior cruciate ligament attachment

sm: Severe pain; variable disability

sg: Swelling; joint effusion; abnormal mobility in anteroposterior plane or upon abduction stress; firm bony block limits knee extension; tenderness not localized over meniscus but beneath patellar tendon

cm: Residual limitation of knee extension; recurrent effusion

xr: Avulsion of tibial spine or of its medial tubercle; or, fracture of lateral tubercle of tibial spine; or, fracture of tibial spine combined with fracture of tibial tuberosity

TIBIA FRACTURE, TUBERCLE AVULSION

at: Patellar Tubercle Fracture Avulsion

et: Fall; running; jumping; stumbling

sm: Local pain; inability to extend knee

sg: Local tenderness and swelling; avulsed fragment palpable, displaced upward with knee flexed

cm: Chronic weakness

xr: Tibial tubercle pulled off, displaced upward

TIBIA FRACTURE, UPPER END

et: Direct blow or crushing injury; indirect violence; fall onto foot with leg bowed outward or inward as margin of tibial condyle is crushed

sm: Pain; inability to bear weight; inability to flex or extend knee voluntarily

sg: Hemarthrosis; effusion; swelling; variable amount of deformity in valgus or varus position; may have deformity in rotation; may have shortening, broadening; tenderness may extend entirely across bone; abnormal mobility of leg outward or inward; false motion in all directions

cm: Traumatic arthritis; residual stiffness; associated injuries

xr: Fracture varies from crack in one condyle without displacement to a transverse fracture of both bones of leg just below knee with vertical splitting and severe comminution of proximal fragment and knee disorganization

TIBIA FRACTURE-SEPARATION, UPPER EPIPHYSIS

at: Tibia Fracture-Separation, Proximal Epiphysis

et: Fall onto feet; excessive forcible abduction or adduction of leg occurs only during adolescence

sm: Pain; disability

sg: Obvious deformity; marked swelling of knee

cm: Injury to popliteal vessels and nerves; growth deformity

xr: Upper tibial epiphysis displaced forward and lateral

TIBIAL CONDYLE OSTEOCHONDRITIS DISSECANS

et: Impingement of articular surfaces; underlying constitutional disorder

sm: Vague pain in joint accentuated by activity and relieved by rest; varying episodes of swelling, locking, or giving way

sg: May palpate loose body; synovial thickening; quadriceps atrophy; crepitus

cm: Persistent disability; traumatic arthritis

xr: Crescentic cavity in medial or lateral tibial condyle with separating of fragment in situ; later, loose body may be seen elsewhere in joint

TINEA CRURIS

at: Jock Itch; Groin Ringworm

et: Fungal infection: epidermophyton floccosum, trichophyton purpureum; heat, humidity, friction of clothing contributory

sm: Pruritus

sg: Superficial, circinate, brownish-red, elevated or macular lesions in intercrural, perineal, gluteal areas; peripheral spread with clearing in center; small satellite lesions; erythema; superficial oozing, crusting

lb: Positive culture

TINEA VERSICOLOR

at: Pityriasis Versicolor; Dermatomycosis Furfuracea; Chromophytosis

et: Infection of skin by malassezia furfur

sm: Mild pruritus

sg: Yellow-brownish macules of epidermis usually of upper trunk, neck, upper abdomen; circumscribed or diffuse lesions

cm: Partial depigmentation following healing

lb: Positive culture from scrapings

TOE DISLOCATION, INTERPHALANGEAL
et: Fall; stubbing toe; direct violence
sm: Pain; disability
sg: Tenderness and swelling about involved toe; ecchymosis; obvious deformity, toe displaced dorsally on proximally adjacent bone
cm: Residual stiffness
xr: Phalanx dislocated dorsally on proximally adjacent bone

TOE FRACTURE, AVULSION
et: Sudden forcible plantarflexion of toe
sm: Pain; disability
sg: Swelling; ecchymosis; tenderness; pain elicited by flexing toe
cm: Tendency for hammer toe deformity to develop
xr: Avulsion fracture of dorsal aspect of base of distal phalanx

TOE FRACTURE, PROXIMAL PHALANX
et: Direct violence; weight falling on foot
sm: Pain; disability
sg: Deformity; false motion; swelling; ecchymosis; crepitus
cm: Residual stiffness
xr: Comminution, longitudinal splitting, transverse or oblique possible

TOE FRACTURE, TIP TUFT
et: Direct violence as from being stepped on
sm: Severe pain at distal end of toe; moderate disability
sg: Subungual hematoma; local swelling, tenderness, ecchymosis; may have deformity
cm: Prolonged disability
xr: Fracture of tuft of tip of distal phalanx

TOE, GREAT, DISLOCATION, INTERPHALANGEAL
et: Stubbing great toe; direct violence
sm: Pain; disability
sg: Obvious deformity; swelling; ecchymosis; tenderness
cm: Residual stiffness
xr: Distal phalanx of great toe displaced dorsally on proximal phalanx; may be displaced medially

TOE, GREAT, DISLOCATION, METATARSOPHALANGEAL
et: Excessive forcible flexion of great toe
sm: Severe pain; disability
sg: Obvious deformity; swelling
cm: Irreducibility; head penetrated plantar part of capsule and may be caught within it or between flexor tendons
xr: Dislocation of metatarsophalangeal joint of great toe; proximal phalanx usually displaced onto dorsum of metatarsal head

TOE, GREAT, FRACTURE, AVULSION
et: Forcible inward thrust on big toe as kicking ball
sm: Pain; disability
sg: Swelling; ecchymosis; tenderness; crepitus
cm: Spurs interfere with dorsiflexion of toe; residual stiffness
xr: Small avulsion fracture, usually involving lateral margin of proximal end of distal or proximal phalanx

TOE, GREAT, FRACTURE, OSTEOCHONDRAL

et: Forceful inward thrust of great toe, as in kicking ball, driving base of either distal or proximal phalanx into opposing head

sm: Severe pain; disability

sg: Swelling; ecchymosis; tenderness; crepitus

cm: Residual stiffness; traumatic arthritis

xr: Osteochondral fracture of head of proximal phalanx or head of first metatarsal with some comminution of base of distal phalanx or base of proximal phalanx

TOE, GREAT, FRACTURE, PHALANX

et: Forceful kick; weight falling on great toe

sm: Throbbing pain over great toe, especially on movement; disability

sg: Local tenderness and swelling; ecchymosis; possible deformity

cm: Residual stiffness; development of spurs

xr: Fracture of phalanx demonstrated; usually not much displacement; may be comminuted, involve joint

TOE, GREAT, FRACTURE, SESAMOIDS

et: Direct violence; fall onto feet; excessive forcible extension of great toe

sm: Pain on hyperextension of great toe and on weight bearing; disability

sg: Local tenderness

cm: Prolonged disability; nonunion

xr: Fracture of sesamoid demonstrated; irregular edges; usually medial sesamoid; rule out bipartite sesamoids

TOE, GREAT, SESAMOIDITIS

et: Excessive forcible dorsiflexion of great toe; direct blow to ball of foot

sm: Persistent severe pain; disability

sg: Tenderness sharply localized under ball of great toe; local swelling

cm: Chronicity

xr: May show bipartite medial sesamoid; transverse separation of the two segments at midline with rounded off margins

TONSILITIS, ACUTE

et: Infection by streptococcus, staphylococcus, other bacteria

sm: Chills, headache, malaise; pain in throat, radiating to ears; dysphagia

sg: High fever; swelling, hyperemia of tonsils; purulent exudate; edema of uvula; cervical lymphadenopathy

cm: Diffuse pharyngitis; peritonsillar abscess; rheumatic fever; acute nephritis

lb: Moderate polymorphonuclear leukocytosis; positive culture from throat smear

TOOTH ABSCESS

at: Periapical Abscess; Dentoalveolar Abscess; Parietal Abscess

et: Chronic periodontitis (parietal abscess); extension of infection from root canal (apical abscess); usually streptococcal

sm: Pain; malaise; may be asymptomatic

sg: Acute suppuration; redness; tooth extrusion; swelling; extreme tenderness to percussion; fever

cm: Granuloma; suppurating osteitis, osteomyelitis, fascial abscess
xr: Diffuse area of radiolucency; well demarcated boundary; acute abscess may not be demonstrated

TOOTH FRACTURE, BREAK

et: Direct trauma; violent occlusion
sm: Local pain
sg: Obvious tooth deformity; one third or more of tooth missing, perhaps including root; often tooth luxation; may have impaired pulp vitality
cm: Pulp necrosis; dental abscess
pa: If limited to incisal or occlusal third, usually does not involve pulp exposure; fracture more cervically generally involves pulp

TOOTH FRACTURE, CHIP

at: Chipped Tooth
et: Direct trauma; violent occlusion
sm: Usually asymptomatic unless tooth luxated
sg: Obvious tooth deformity; small piece of tooth missing

TOOTH FRACTURE, LINEAR

at: Cracked Tooth
et: Unknown; direct trauma; violent occlusion
sm: Local pain, especially on occlusion
sg: Tenderness on percussion; linear crack, usually longitudinal; may have impaired pulp vitality
cm: Pulp necrosis; dental abscess
pa: If limited to incisal or occlusal third, usually does not involve pulp exposure; fracture more cervically generally involves pulp

TOOTH FRACTURE, ROOT

et: Direct Trauma
sm: Local pain, especially on occlusion
sg: Mobility, varying with location of fracture; injury to supporting structure
cm: Pulp necrosis; dental abscess
xr: Fracture of root demonstrated

TOOTH, INTRUDED

et: Direct trauma to long axis of tooth
sm: Local pain
sg: Local tenderness, swelling; displacement apically into socket from functional occlusal plane
cm: Pulp devitalization; root resorption; eventual loss of tooth
xr: May show root or tooth in antrum

TOOTH, LUXATED, COMPLETE

at: Missing Tooth; Completely Displaced Tooth
et: Direct trauma
sm: Severe pain
sg: Dislocation of tooth from socket; bleeding; swelling
cm: Osteomyelitis; eventual extrusion of opposing tooth

TOOTH, LUXATED, PARTIAL

at: Loose Tooth
et: Direct trauma; violent malocclusion
sm: Local pain, instability of tooth
sg: Tooth loose in socket; tenderness on percussion; possible swelling of peridontium
cm: Subsequent malocclusion; extraction

TROCHANTERIC BURSITIS

et: Direct blow; contusion of greater trochanter; infection; friction between adjacent bursal walls overlying greater trochanter
sm: Pain; varying disability
sg: Local tenderness; crepitus; pain elicited by forcible activity of thigh
xr: Occasional calcification within bursal sac

TUBERCULOSIS, PULMONARY

et: Mycobacterium tuberculosis
sm: Gradual onset; malaise; fatigue; loss of weight; chills; cough; dyspnea; hoarseness; nocturnal sweats; hemoptysis; thoracic pain
sg: Onset may be pneumonic; slight elevation of fever late in afternoon, increasing and subsiding in recurrent episodes; delayed expansion of chest over affected area; impairment of pulmonary resonance; rales; pleural friction-rub
cm: Pleurisy with effusion; empyema; pneumothorax; atelectasis; laryngeal tuberculosis; extension to other organs, regions; pulmonary impairment
lb: Positive culture of sputum smear; positive tuberculin test
xr: Variable; striations; areas of increased density; calcification; thickening of pleura; enlargement of mediastinal lymph nodes
pa: Fibroulcerative, fibrocavitary lesions in apical, subapical, lower lobe of lung

ULNA FRACTURE, CENTRAL THIRD

et: Direct blow
sm: Pain; disability
sg: Swelling; tenderness; possible deformity
cm: Impairment of pronation, supination; nonunion
xr: Fracture of central ulna shaft demonstrated; possibly displacement

ULNA FRACTURE, DISTAL THIRD

et: Direct or indirect trauma
sm: Pain; disability
sg: Swelling; tenderness; crepitus; possible deformity; false motion
xr: Fracture of lower ulna shaft demonstrated; possibly displacement

ULNA FRACTURE, OLECRANON

at: Elbow Fracture
et: Direct blow as in fall onto elbow; avulsion of olecranon by violent contraction of triceps muscle; fall onto semiflexed and supinated forearm
sm: Pain; disability
sg: Swelling; crepitus; gap between fragments or alteration in relationship between process and epicondyles palpable; inability to flex or

extend elbow

xr: Fracture line of olecranon in transverse direction, extending into joint; variable degree of separation of fragments

ULNA FRACTURE, PROXIMAL THIRD
et: Direct blow
sm: Pain; disability
sg: Swelling; deformity; tenderness; crepitus
xr: Fracture of upper ulna shaft demonstrated; usually posterior displacement of fragment

ULNAR NERVE DISLOCATION, RECURRENT
et: Unknown; trauma; shallow ulnar groove on humeral medial epicondyle predisposing
sm: Pain and sensation of something slipping back of elbow during flexion-extension of joint; warmness and tingling over inner border of hand; recurrent disability
sg: Tenderness of nerve in ulnar groove at elbow; excessive mobility of nerve on palpation, may be dislocated painfully; sensory changes in hand; weakness, atrophy of small muscles of hand
cm: Ulnar palsy
pa: Inflammation and thickening of nerve sheath at elbow strangling enclosed fibers

URTICARIA, NONALLERGENIC
et: Release of histamine from mast cells into blood stream, acting on blood vessel; predisposing agents: codeine, atrophine, parasites, environmental stress reactions, psychogenic stress, exertional stress, skin disease
sm: Pruritus, pricking sensation during early formation of fluid in wheals; abdominal pain; hoarseness with mucosal involvement
sg: Transient erythematous or whitish swellings in skin; wheals; oval and round lesions, enlarging by peripheral extension becoming confluent
cm: Edema of larynx; anaphylactic shock
lb: Cutaneous testing in chronic cases of virtually no value

VAGINITIS
et: Trichomonas; monilia; usually, mixed bacterial infection
sm: Vaginal discharge; pruritus and irritation of vulvae
sg: White, yellow, or greenish discharge; inflamed vulvar area and vagina; commonly with cervical erosion
cm: Endometritis
lb: Hanging wet drop slide reveals trichomonas; smear and culture reveals monilia

VARICOCELE
et: Unknown; venous valvular incompetence
sm: Usually asymptomatic; pain in area of scrotum; dull pulling, dragging sensation disappearing in supine position; exacerbations with hernia, venous thromboses
sg: Mass of veins in scrotum palpable in standing position; bluish appearance through scrotal skin; disappear in recumbent position

VERTEBRA, TRANSITIONAL
et: Congenital; less stable than normal back, and more inclined through faulty mechanics and trauma to develop ligamentous and muscular involvement

sm: May be asymptomatic; low back pain especially after exertion or prolonged standing; radiating leg pain

sg: Decreased lumbosacral motion; paravertebral muscle spasm and tenderness

cm: Chronic disability

xr: Sacralization of last lumbar vertebra; one or both transverse processes of last lumbar vertebra is long and wingshaped, and either articulates with or is fused to sacrum and/or ilium; more often bilateral; or, persistence of first sacral segment as a separate vertebra

VERTEBRAL ARTERY OCCLUSION

et: Sudden forcible cervical hyperextension injury; vertebral artery compressed between occipital condyles and first cervical vertebra laminae or between C1 and C2 vertebrae upon their dislocation

sm: If thrombosed: immediate unconsciousness, tetraplegia and/or death. If spasm: inability to move hands, arms, and probably legs but movement of toes; rapid recovery

sg: If thrombosed: inability to rouse, tetraplegia, gradual or immediate respiratory failure. If spasm: paralysis in upper extremities and paresis in lower ones but movement of toes; gradual clearing; may have no sensory loss; rapid recovery

cm: Basilar artery thrombosis secondary to ascending vertebral artery thrombosis; death

xr: If thrombosis: atlantoaxial dislocation may be present. If spasm: no fracture. CAUTION: direct angiography may produce respiratory failure or tetraplegia

pa: Thrombosis or spasm occludes lumen

VERTEBRAL EPIPHYSITIS, DORSAL

at: Scheuerman's Disease; Juvenile Kyphosis; Adolescent Roundback; Vertebral Osteochondritis

et: Unknown; usually begins at 13-16 years of age

sm: Pain in thoracic spine, subsiding after several months

sg: Rounded back, slight or moderate thoracic kyphosis; in active stage, tenderness on firm palpation over site

cm: May be disabling in acute or later stage; osteoarthritic lipping of anterior vertebral margin; permanent wedging of affected vertebrae

lb: Erythrocyte sedimentation rate not raised

xr: Active stage: affected vertebral bodies show deep notched defects at anterior corners; corresponding parts of ring epiphyses may be irregular in size and shape; disc spaces are slightly narrowed but never totally destroyed. After healing: slight anteroposterior wedging of affected vertebral bodies

pa: Disturbance of normal development of cartilage plates and ring epiphyses, possibly from bursting of disc contents through cartilage into subjacent vertebral body

WART

at: Verruca

et: Viral infection; epidermal thickening

sm: Possible pain on pressure

sg: Single or multiple small round elevated lesions with rough, dry surfaces; usually sessile; completely ectopic, affecting skin, mucosa adjacent to mucocutaneous junctions; unpredictable course

lb: Filterable infectious agent in tissue

pa: Papillary acanthosis surrounded by friable keratotic material; usually focally pigmented with fine brown granules of melanin

115

WOLFF-PARKINSON-WHITE SYNDROME

at: Anomalous Atrioventricular Excitation
et: Congenital; conduction over aberrant bundle of cardiac muscle by-passing normal auriculoventricular bundle, causing premature activation of portion of ventricular musculature; acceleration in conduction through fibers of AV node
sm: Episodes of paroxysmal tachycardia beginning in youth
lb: EKG demonstrates normal P waves, short P-R interval, increased duration of QRS

WOUND, HUMAN BITE

et: Laceration resulting from forcible contact with another's teeth as in involvement of knuckle from punch
sm: Local pain; bleeding
sg: Open, ragged wound
cm: Serious deep infection from mouth organisms; suppurative arthritis; osteomyelitis
xr: Fragment of fractured tooth may be demonstrated

WOUND, PENETRATING

at: Includes: Puncture Wound; Stab Wound; Cleat Wound
et: Penetration by object or missile such as javelin, nail, cleat
sm: Local pain
sg: Variable, depending on site and severity; bleeding; open or closed wound; tenderness; shock
cm: Infection, such as tetanus

WRIST SPRAIN, HYPEREXTENSION

at: Dorsiflexion Wrist Sprain
et: Fall onto outstretched hand; excessive forcible pressure against palm of hand
sm: Pain over dorsal and volar aspect of wrist, especially on motion; weakness
sg: Grade by degree of severity: swelling; tenderness
xr: Fracture ruled out, especially navicular fracture

WRIST SPRAIN, HYPERFLEXION

at: Volar Flexion Wrist Sprain
et: Fall onto volar flexed hand
sm: Pain over dorsum of wrist, especially on motion; weakness
sg: Grade by degree of severity: swelling; tenderness
xr: Fracture ruled out

ZYGOMA FRACTURE

at: Malar Fracture
et: Direct blow as from punch, baseball, hockey puck
sm: Pain; numbness of lip; difficulty in opening, closing mouth; diplopia, other disturbances varying with associated injuries
sg: External evidence of trauma to cheek; swelling; edema, possibly involving eyelids; cheek asymmetry; emphysema of cheek; nasal bleeding; other irregularities varying with associated injuries
cm: Permanent deformity; permanent anesthesia of upper lip; possible visual impairment from associated orbit fracture

xr: Modified Waters' position shows lesions best; planigrams helpful; fracture demonstrated at zygoma articulations; frequently associated with fractures of maxilla and zygomatic process; orbit blowout fracture also may be present

ZYGOMATIC ARCH FRACTURE

et: Direct blow; indirect trauma secondary to displaced fracture of zygoma

sm: Pain, discomfort in talking or chewing

sg: Depression deformity, perhaps prominence, at fracture site; swelling; tenderness; irregularity or fracture displacement palpable

xr: Submental-occipital view demonstrates fracture, usually in three places: at each end and in middle of arch; usually medial displacement

cm: Impingement of coronoid process of mandible and temporalis muscle

GLOSSARY

ABDUCTION   The act of drawing a body segment away from the median line of a proximally conjoined segment

ADDUCTION   The act of drawing a body segment toward the median line of a proximally conjoined segment

ALBUMINURIA, ORTHOSTATIC (Postural Albuminuria)
Presence of albumin in urine when subject stands or sits; disappears upon reclining; not related to demonstrable pathology

AMENORRHEA   Absence or abnormal stoppage of the menses

ANAPHYLAXIS   A spectacular tissue allergenic reaction developing from a few minutes to a half hour following an injection of an antigen or sting of an insect to which sensitization is present; chief manifestations are collapse, asthma, fainting, urticaria, convulsions, lessened coagulability of the blood, coma, and death

ANKYLOSIS   Permanent consolidation, restriction of joint motion from abnormal fibrous or bony overgrowth

ARRHYTHMIA, SINUS   Variation in rhythm of heart beat dependent on interference with the impulses originating in the sinoauricular node; not associated with disease but with inspiration and expiration

ATHLETE'S HEART   Normal, healthy, efficient heart in well-conditioned athlete; apparent enlargement on silhouette may be from ventricular hypertrophy and/or increased distensibility; returns to prior size after cessation of training

119

*AURA   Premonitory symptom prior to onset of a seizure as recognized by subject

BLOCKER'S DISEASE   The development of a bony growth at the middle third of the arm at or near the insertion of the deltoid from repeated contusions to that site; whether this complication is termed an exostosis or traumatic myositis ossificans depends on whether the bony formation has or has not infiltrated through the muscle tissue

BRADYCARDIA   Unusually slow heart beat ranging from 40-60 beats per minute; nonpathologic if due to increased heart efficiency from endurance training

BUNIONETTE   Bony enlargement of lateral side of head of 5th metatarsal at the metatarsophalangeal joint; associated with an overlying bursal sac and a medial deviation of 5th toe

CALCIUM DEPOSIT   Abnormal calcification of soft tissue from traumatic insult, usually repeated episodes

*CONFUSION   Trauma-produced mental state in which reactions to environmental stimuli are inappropriate

*CONSCIOUSNESS   A state of general wakefulness and responsiveness to one's environment; impairment of consciousness, short of unconsciousness, is commonly described with no unanimity of precise meaning as lethargy, stupor, coma, and semiconsciousness

CONVULSION   Seizure with or without unconsciousness which may or may not be associated with various sensory or motor components described under epilepsy

COTTONMOUTH   Sensation of discomfort associated with dry mouth from dehydration or emotional tension

DELIRIUM, POST-TRAUMATIC   Form of post-traumatic neuropsychological disorder, displaying disturbed consciousness, agitation, hallucinations, delusions and/or disorientation.

*DEMENTIA, POST-TRAUMATIC   Form of post-traumatic neuropsychological disorder, displaying mental impairment

DIARRHEA   Evacuation of loose or watery stools from any of many causes including pathogenic microorganisms, emotional state, and various conditions and diseases of the gastrointestinal tract

DORSIFLEXION   The act of drawing the toe or foot, finger or wrist, toward the dorsal aspect of the proximally conjoined body segment

DRYING OUT   Practice of purposeful dehydration for artificial weight control

120

DYSPEPSIA (Indigestion)   Symptom-complex including nausea, heartburn, flatulence, eructations; emotional tension or food incompatibility may produce symptoms, but underlying organic disease sometimes present

ECCHYMOSIS   General extravasation of blood in soft tissues from blow producing skin discoloration

EPISTAXIS (Nose Bleed)   Hemorrhage emanating from tissues of nasal cavity

ERYTHEMA   Superficial congestion of capillaries causing surface redness, warmth

EVERSION   The act of rotating the pronated foot externally on the ankle

EXOSTOSIS   Localized benign bony overgrowth

EXTENSION   The act of drawing a body segment toward a straight line position with its proximally conjoined body segment

FLEXION   The act of drawing a body segment away from a straight line with its proximally conjoined body segment or toward that joint's smallest acute angle

FRACTURE   Breaking of continuity of bone or cartilage

FRACTURE, ANGULATION   Fracture in which fragments are moved out of a linear relationship into an angular relationship

FRACTURE, AVULSION   Fracture in which fragment of bone avulses at attachment of tendon, ligament, or muscle, secondary to sudden violent stress; avulsion is incidental to the sprain or strain that occurred

FRACTURE, CHONDRAL   Fracture involving articular cartilage only

FRACTURE, CLOSED   Fracture in which there is no wound extending from the surface to the site of bony injury

FRACTURE, COMMINUTED   Fracture in which three or more fragments are produced

FRACTURE, COMPLETE   Fracture in which bone continuity is completely interrupted

FRACTURE, COMPRESSION   Impacted fracture characterized by crushed bone tissue

FRACTURE, DELAYED UNION   Fracture which has not united successfully within expected period of time

FRACTURE, DISPLACED   Fracture in which bone fragment
is out of its normal alignment

FRACTURE, FATIGUE (March Fracture, Stress Fracture)
Fracture occurring after prolonged repetitive activity against firm resistance; no history of specific traumatic incident

FRACTURE, GREENSTICK   Incomplete fracture of long
bone shaft in which cortex is broken on convexity of curve while bone on
concave surface is bent; split usually longitudinal in either direction from
fracture site

FRACTURE, IMPACTED   Fracture in which one fragment
has been driven into and embedded in another fragment

FRACTURE, INCOMPLETE   Fracture in which bone continuity is not completely interrupted

FRACTURE, MALUNION   Fracture which has united with
faulty alignment of fragments

FRACTURE, NONUNION (Ununited Fracture)   Fracture
which has not repaired in bony union

FRACTURE, OBLIQUE   Fracture in which the break extends
in an oblique direction

FRACTURE, OPEN (Compound Fracture)   Fracture in
which an open wound extends through the skin and down to the site of
the bony injury; primary type is that which occurs at time of fracture;
secondary type is that which is opened by surgery or sloughing of tissue
over fracture site

FRACTURE, OSTEOCHONDRAL   Fracture involving articular cartilage and underlying bone

FRACTURE, OVERRIDING   Fracture in which fragments
overlap, resulting in shortening of bone

FRACTURE, PATHOLOGICAL   Fracture occurring through
an area which has been previously weakened by disease or tumor; usually
occurs following minimal trauma

FRACTURE, ROTATED   Fracture in which one fragment has
rotated on its axis in relation to other

FRACTURE, SPIRAL   Fracture with spiral fracture line occurring in long bones from a twisting injury

FRACTURE-DISLOCATION   Fracture near a joint at which
dislocation occurs concurrently from same traumatic incident

122

FUNNY BONE (Crazy Bone)   Contusion of ulnar nerve at the ulnar groove of the humeral medial epicondyle producing a transiently disabling burning sensation and numbness along ulnar side of forearm and hand

GANGRENE   Anemic necrosis of tissue; combined usually with invasion of saphrophytic organisms

GENU RECURVATUM   Hyperextensibility of knee; usually congenital in origin; may be predisposing factor in internal derangement of knee

GENU VALGUM (Knock-knee)   Deformity, usually congenital, but may be secondary to trauma; knees abnormally close together while the space between ankles is increased; curvature of leg with apex of convexity displaced medially at level of knee; may be predisposing factor in development of recurrent subluxation or dislocation of patella, or of medial collateral ligament sprain

HALLUX RIGIDUS   Osteoarthritis of metatarsophalangeal joint of great toe with marked restriction of motion; x-ray film shows narrowing of cartilage space, subchondral sclerosis, and spurring or lipping of joint margins

HALLUX VALGUS   Lateral deviation of great toe at metatarsophalangeal joint

HEADACHE   Symptom of head pain; variable in duration, intensity, and site; cause may be from trauma, tension, disease, tumor, dehydration, or unknown factors

HEART BURN   Burning sensation over heart area but coming from esophagus or stomach; related to reflux of gastric contents; frequently of functional origin but organic cause may be present; nervousness, faulty digestion contributory

HEART MURMUR   Atypical heart sound(s); may be functional and of no clinical significance; or, may be indicative of pathological valvular lesions requiring clinical attention

HEAT FATIGUE   Transient deterioration in performance from exposure to heat, humidity, and resulting in relative state of dehydration and salt depletion.

HEMARTHROSIS   Blood extravasated into joint

HEMATOMA   Pooling of extravasated blood within tissues or organs

HEMATURIA, MICROSCOPIC   Blood in urine; occurs in most sports that require marked exertion or with frequent trauma; distinguish from gross hematuria which reflects more serious damage to genitourinary system

123

HEMOPTYSIS   Act of coughing up blood; caused by lesion of lungs, trachea, or larynx

HOT SPOT   Early redness of skin from friction that leads to blister formation if preventive measures not taken

HYPERTENSION, LABILE   Unstable blood pressure characteristically elevated during periods of nervous tension and subsiding with rest

HYPHEMA   Hemorrhage into anterior chamber of eye fellowing trauma

HYPOGLYCEMIA   Blood glucose level below normal

INVERSION   The act of rotating the supinated foot medially on the ankle

KNEE, INTERNAL DERANGEMENT   Traumatic injury to knee in which lesions are produced in any of the internal structures comprising the joint's integrity: menisci, cruciate ligaments, tibial spine, articular cartilages, infrapatellar fat pad

KNEE, ROTARY INSTABILITY   Abnormal external rotation of tibia on femur due to tear of the knee's medial capsule; characterized by the athlete's inability to change direction sharply (although his ability to run forward is unimpaired) subsequent to a forced abduction and external rotation injury of a flexed knee

LACE BITE   Painful inflammation over dorsum of foot, usually over prominent ridge of base of first metatarsal; develops usually from abrasive irritation of tightly laced footwear

MENORRHAGIA   Excessive or prolonged menstruation due to disorders of endocrine, generative, or circulatory systems, acute infectious diseases, blood dyscrasia, emotional or environmental factors

METRORRHAGIA   Abnormal uterine hemorrhage, especially during intermenstrual period

MUSCLE ATROPHY   Wasting away of muscle tissue as the result of immobilization (casts), inactivity, loss of innervation, or nutritional disorder

MUSCLE CRAMP   Painful involuntary contraction of skeletal muscle group; causes include salt depletion (heat cramp), fatigue, and reflex reaction to trauma

MYOPIA (Nearsightedness)   Defective eyesight due to refractive error in the eye causing rays from distant objects to focus in front of retina

NAUSEA   Sensation of distention and/or discomfort in region of stomach often followed by vomiting; numerous causes; psychogenic, overeating, food intolerance, local disease, reaction to systemic disease or condition, manifestation of drug toxicity

NEAR-DROWNING   A critical aquatic predicament resolved by successful water rescue

OSTEOARTHRITIS   Degeneration of articular cartilage from congenital, traumatic, inflammatory, and/or aging factors

PARAPLEGIA   Extensive loss of neural function, both sensory and motor, below level of lesion of spinal cord at or below level of first thoracic vertebra

PATELLA BIPARTITE   Failure of patellar ossification center to fuse in superolateral corner, thus producing two parts; usually bilateral, symmetrical; usually asymptomatic

PES CAVUS (Hollow Foot)   Accentuated high longitudinal arch; may be congenital or result from neurological disorder causing muscular imbalance; clawing of toes always associated and shortening of achilles tendon frequently present; as a result, excessive weight is placed on metatarsal heads, calluses develop in the underlying skin

PINCHED NERVE SYNDROME (Nerve Contusion)
Term used to describe transient root-like pain and other manifestations resulting from injury to the neck as in blocking and tackling (See nerve contusion; overriding articular facets; ruptured disc.)

PLANTARFLEXION   The act of drawing the toe or foot toward the plantar aspect of the proximally conjoined body segment

POST-CONCUSSION SYNDROME   Persistent variable symptoms of headache, tinnitus, dizziness, and/or confusion subsequent to a cerebral concussive incident

PRONATION   The act of rotating a hand or foot internally on its long axis

PRURITUS ANI   Intractable itching in anal area often due to unknown cause; may be associated with local infection, hemorrhoids, or other local conditions; poor anal hygiene contributory; possibly allergy, emotional and tension states

SEPTICEMIA   Presence of pathogenic organisms and their toxins in circulatory system

SEPTUM, DEVIATED   Post-traumatic or congenitally deformed nasal septum causing a degree of nasal passage obstruction

SHIN SPLINTS   Pain and discomfort in leg from repetitive running on hard surface or forcible excessive use of foot flexors; diagnosis should be limited to musculotendinous inflammations, excluding fatigue fracture or ischemic disorder

SHOCK   A critical clinical condition characterized by variable signs and symptoms which arise when the cardiac output is insufficient to fill the arterial tree with blood under sufficient pressure to provide organs and tissues with adequate blood flow; often present with severe trauma and hemorrhage

SPEARING   Act of butting head into midsection or chest of opponent; hazardous to spearer (cervical spine injury) as well as to opponent (direct trauma)

STALE (Slump)   A psychological or physiological state of overtraining which manifests as deteriorated athletic readiness

SUPINATION   The act of rotating a hand or foot externally on its long axis

SYNCOPE (Fainting)   A mild and transient form of shock with a short period of unconsciousness from which rapid recovery is made upon assuming a horizontal position; in the emotional or psychogenic type, vasovagal reflexes slow the heart and bring on peripheral vasodilatation, thereby diminishing cardiac output.

SYNOVITIS, TRAUMATIC   Painful inflammation of the synovial membrane (inner lining) of a joint secondary to injury; characterized by the development of fluid within the joint (synovial effusion), perhaps mixed with blood (hemarthrosis)

TAPE BURN   Skin rash at site of tape application due to mechanical effects or allergy

TENDON DISLOCATION   Displacement of tendon from its normal position in a groove over bony fulcrum or neighboring soft tissue

TETRAPLEGIA (Quadriplegia)   Motor and sensory loss in all four extremities from spinal cord lesion at cervical level

TINNITUS   The sensation of a ringing in ears from traumatic or other causes

TOE, HAMMER (Hallux Malleus)   Fixed flexion deformity of proximal interphalangeal joint of toe with compensatory hyperextension of distal interphalangeal joint; callus forms over dorsum of flexed joint from pressure against shoe

TOOTH EXTRUSION Frequent type of displacement of deciduous and/or permanent teeth; tooth moves beyond functional occlusal plane because of lack of resisting pressure against extracted or malaligned tooth

TRIAD, UNHAPPY Classic injury in football resulting from being blocked on lateral side of knee with foot fixed to ground; inward rotation of thigh on an externally rotated leg accompanying the lateral stress produces medial collateral sprain, medial meniscus tear, and anterior cruciate sprain

TRIGGER POINT A focal point of irritation which when stimulated sets off a painful reaction referred to a distant area or areas

*UNCONSCIOUSNESS Loss of wakefulness and responsiveness to one's environment

VARICOSE VEINS Dilatation of superficial veins, usually in leg, from valvular incompetency producing pain, discomfort

VOLAR FLEXION The act of drawing the fingers or hand toward the palmar aspect of the proximally conjoined body segment

*WHIPLASH Popular term for hyperextension-hyperflexion injury to cervical spine; does not imply any specific resultant pathology

UNACCEPTABLE TERMS

The following terms are representative of commonly used colloquialisms perpetuating confusion and impreciseness in athletic medicine terminology. Such terms are not recommended because of their nonspecificity and widespread variation in meaning. The reader is encouraged to substitute preferred terminology found in the text of this publication.

BASKETBALL KNEE

BELLRUNG

CATCH

CRICK

DEAD ARM

FOOTBALL KNEE

FOOTBALL SHOULDER

FROG

GLASS ARM

KINK

KNOCKED DOWN SHOULDER

PITCHER'S ELBOW

RIB OUT

RUPTURE

SEPARATION

TENNIS LEG

TRICK KNEE

CROSS-INDEX OF TERMS

All terms in capital letters are preferred terms to be located alphabetically in the text or glossary (gl)

ABDUCTION (gl)

ABRASION

ABSCESS

ABSCESS, AXILLARY

Abscess, Collar Button: ABSCESS, PALMAR SPACE

ABSCESS, PALMAR SPACE

Abscess, Tooth: TOOTH ABSCESS

Abscess, Web-Space: ABSCESS, PALMAR SPACE

ACCESSORY TARSAL NAVICULAR FRACTURE

ACETABULUM FRACTURE

ACETABULUM FRACTURE, CHONDRAL

ACHILLES TENDON STRAIN

ACHILLES TENDON TENOSYNOVITIS

ACHILLOBURSITIS

ACNE VULGARIS

acromial, Sub-, Bursitis: SUBACROMIAL BURSITIS

Acromioclavicular Dislocation: ACROMIOCLAVICULAR SPRAIN, 3RD DEGREE

Acromioclavicular Separation: ACROMIOCLAVICULAR SPRAIN, 2ND DEGREE

ACROMIOCLAVICULAR SPRAIN, 1ST DEGREE

ACROMIOCLAVICULAR SPRAIN, 2ND DEGREE

ACROMIOCLAVICULAR SPRAIN, 3RD DEGREE

ADDUCTION (gl)

ADDUCTOR LONGUS STRAIN

ADDUCTOR MAGNUS STRAIN

ALBUMINURIA, ORTHOSTATIC (gl)

Albuminuria, Postural: ALBUMINURIA, ORTHOSTATIC (gl)

Alkalosis, Respiratory: HYPERVENTILATION SYNDROME

AMENORRHEA (gl)

ANAL FISSURE

ANAPHYLAXIS (gl)

Aneurysm, Berry: ANEURYSM, CEREBRAL

ANEURYSM, CEREBRAL

Angioedema, Circumscribed: ANGIONEUROTIC EDEMA

ANGIONEUROTIC EDEMA

Angulation Fracture: FRACTURE, ANGULATION (gl)

Ani Pruritus: PRURITUS, ANI (gl)

Ankle, Chipped: ANKLE FRACTURE, LATERAL or MEDIAL MALLEOLUS AVULSION

ANKLE DISLOCATION, ANTERIOR

ANKLE DISLOCATION, POSTERIOR

ANKLE DISLOCATION, UPWARD

ANKLE EXOSTOSES, TALOTIBIAL

ANKLE FRACTURE, ABDUCTION, 1ST DEGREE

ANKLE FRACTURE, ABDUCTION, 2ND DEGREE

ANKLE FRACTURE, ABDUCTION, 3RD DEGREE

ANKLE FRACTURE, ADDUCTION, 1ST DEGREE

ANKLE FRACTURE, ADDUCTION, 2ND DEGREE

ANKLE FRACTURE, ADDUCTION, 3RD DEGREE

ANKLE FRACTURE, EXTERNAL ROTATION, 1ST DEGREE

ANKLE FRACTURE, EXTERNAL ROTATION, 2ND DEGREE

ANKLE FRACTURE, EXTERNAL ROTATION, 3RD DEGREE

ANKLE FRACTURE, LATERAL MALLEOLUS AVULSION

ANKLE FRACTURE, MEDIAL MALLEOLUS AVULSION

ANKLE FRACTURE-SEPARATION, DISTAL TIBIOFIBULAR EPIPHYSES

ANKLE SPRAIN, DELTOID LIGAMENT

Ankle Sprain, Eversion: ANKLE SPRAIN, DELTOID LIGAMENT

ANKLE SPRAIN, FIBULAR COLLATERAL LIGAMENT

Ankle Sprain, Inversion: ANKLE SPRAIN, FIBULAR COLLATERAL LIGAMENT

Ankle Sprain, Lateral Collateral Ligament: ANKLE SPRAIN, FIBULAR COLLATERAL LIGAMENT

Ankle Sprain, Medial Collateral Ligament: ANKLE SPRAIN, DELTOID LIGAMENT

Ankle Sprain-Fracture, Eversion: ANKLE FRACTURE, MEDIAL MALLEOLUS AVULSION

Ankle Sprain-Fracture, Inversion: ANKLE FRACTURE, LATERAL MALLEOLUS AVULSION

Ankle Spur: ANKLE EXOSTOSES, TALOTIBIAL

ANKLE SUBLUXATION, RECURRENT

ANKYLOSIS (gl)

ANSERINE BURSITIS

ANTERIOR TIBIAL COMPARTMENT SYNDROME

ANTERIOR TIBIAL TENDON TENOSYNOVITIS

ANXIETY REACTION

Aorta, Aortic Valve: see HEART, . . .

APOCRINITIS

APPENDICITIS, ACUTE

ARCH SPRAIN, STATIC

ARCH SPRAIN, TRAUMATIC

Arches, Fallen: FLATFEET, SYMPTOMATIC

ARRHYTHMIA, SINUS (gl)

Artery Occlusion, Internal Carotid: INTERNAL CAROTID ARTERY OCCLUSION

Artery Occlusion, Vertebral: VERTEBRAL ARTERY OCCLUSION

Arthritis, Purulent: ARTHRITIS, SUPPURATIVE

Arthritis, Pyogenic: ARTHRITIS, SUPPURATIVE

Arthritis, Septic: ARTHRITIS, SUPPURATIVE

Arthritis, Spinal Atrophic: SPONDYLITIS, RHEUMATOID

ARTHRITIS, SUPPURATIVE

ARTHRITIS, TRAUMATIC

ASTHMA, BRONCHIAL

Astragalus: see TALUS

ATHLETE'S FOOT

ATHLETE'S HEART (gl)

Atlantoaxial Dislocation: SPINE DISLOCATION, ATLANTOAXIAL

Atrioventricular Excitation, Anomalous: WOLFF-PARKINSON-WHITE SYNDROME

Atrophy, Muscle: MUSCLE ATROPHY (gl)

AURA (gl)

Avulsion Fracture: FRACTURE, AVULSION (gl)

Axillary Abscess: ABSCESS, AXILLARY

Baker's Cyst: POPLITEAL CYST

BARTON FRACTURE

BASEBALL FINGER

BENNETT'S FRACTURE

Berry Aneurysm: ANEURYSM, CEREBRAL

BICIPITAL TENOSYNOVITIS

Bite Wound: WOUND, HUMAN BITE

Black Eye: PERIORBITAL HEMATOMA

Blackhead: ACNE VULGARIS

BLISTER, FRICTION

BLOCKER'S DISEASE (gl)

Blowout Fracture: ORBIT BLOWOUT FRACTURE

Boil: FURUNCULOSIS

Bone Bruise: PERIOSTITIS, TRAUMATIC; or, FOOT CONTUSION, PLANTAR

BONE CYST, SOLITARY

BONE DEFECT, FIBROUS METAPHYSEAL

BONE FIBROMA, NONOSTEOGENIC

Bone Infection, Acute: OSTEOMYELITIS, ACUTE

BONE TUMOR, GIANT CELL
BOUTONNIERRE DEFORMITY
Boxer's Fracture: METACARPAL FRACTURE, NECK
Buttonhole Deformity: BOUTONNIERRE DEFORMITY
BRACHIAL PLEXUS STRETCH INJURY
BRADYCARDIA (gl)
BRAIN SYNDROME, CHRONIC
BRONCHITIS, ACUTE
Bruise: CONTUSION
BUNION
BUNIONETTE (gl)
BURN, CHEMICAL
BURN, 1ST DEGREE
BURN, 2ND DEGREE
BURN, 3RD DEGREE
BURSITIS
CALCANEAL APOPHYSIS AVULSION
CALCANEAL APOPHYSITIS
calcaneal, Retro-, Bursitis, Superficial: ACHILLOBURSITIS
CALCANEOCUBOID LIGAMENT SPRAIN
CALCANEUS FRACTURE, BODY
CALCANEUS FRACTURE, MARGIN AVULSION
CALCANEUS FRACTURE, SUSTENTACULUM TALI
CALCANEUS FRACTURE, TUBEROSITY AVULSION
CALCIUM DEPOSIT (gl)
CALF STRAIN
Callosity: CALLUS
CALLUS
Candida Albicans: MONILIASIS, CUTANEOUS
CARBUNCLE
Caries: DENTAL CARIES
CARPAL NAVICULAR FRACTURE
CARPOMETACARPAL, FIRST, DISLOCATION
Carpometacarpal, First, Fracture-Dislocation: BENNETT FRACTURE
CARPOMETACARPAL SUBLUXATION
Catarrhal Fever: INFLUENZA
CAUDA EQUINA CONCUSSION
CAUDA EQUINA CONTUSION
Cauliflower Ear: EAR, CAULIFLOWER
CELIAC PLEXUS SYNDROME
CELLULITIS

132

Cellulitis, Finger: FELON

Cerebral Aneurysm: ANEURYSM, CEREBRAL

CEREBRAL CONCUSSION, ACUTE, 1ST DEGREE

CEREBRAL CONCUSSION, ACUTE, 2ND DEGREE

CEREBRAL CONCUSSION, ACUTE, 3RD DEGREE

Cerebral Concussion, Mild: CEREBRAL CONCUSSION, ACUTE, 1ST DEGREE

Cerebral Concussion, Moderate: CEREBRAL CONCUSSION, ACUTE, 2ND DEGREE

Cerebral Concussion, Severe: CEREBRAL CONCUSSION, ACUTE, 3RD DEGREE

Cerebral Hemorrhage, Extradural: CRANIOCEREBRAL HEMATOMA, EPIDURAL

CEREBRAL HEMORRHAGE, SUBARACHNOID

Cerebral Hemorrhage, Subdural: CRANIOCEREBRAL HEMATOMA, SUBDURAL

cerebral, Intra-, Clot, Hematoma or Hemorrhage: INTRACEREBRAL HEMORRHAGE

CEREBRAL HYDROMA, SUBDURAL

Cerebral Hydroma, Subdural: CEREBRAL HYDROMA, SUBDURAL

Cerebral Injury, Chronic: BRAIN SYNDROME, CHRONIC

Cervical Arthritis, Traumatic: SPONDYLOSIS, CERVICAL

Cervical Disc Rupture: DISC RUPTURE, CERVICAL

Cervical Spondylosis: SPONDYLOSIS, CERVICAL

CERVICAL SPINE SPRAIN

Cervical Syndrome: SPINAL CORD SYNDROME, ACUTE, ANTERIOR or CENTRAL CERVICAL

Cervical Vertebra Dislocation, Articular Process: SPINE DISLOCATION, CERVICAL ARTICULAR PROCESS

Cervical Vertebra Facets, Locked, Overriding: SPINE DISLOCATION, CERVICAL ARTICULAR PROCESS

Cervical Vertebra Fracture, Axial Arch Avulsion: SPINE FRACTURE, HANGMAN'S

Cervical Vertebra Fracture, Explosive: SPINE FRACTURE, TEARDROP

Cervical Vertebra, Jumped Process Complex: SPINE DISLOCATION, CERVICAL ARTICULAR PROCESS

Chafing: INTERTRIGO

CHARLEYHORSE

Cheek Fracture: ZYGOMA FRACTURE

Chondral Fracture: FRACTURE, CHONDRAL (gl)

CHONDROSARCOMA

Chromophytosis: TINEA VERSICOLOR

Cinderburn: ABRASION

CLAVICLE FRACTURE, INNER THIRD

CLAVICLE FRACTURE, MIDDLE THIRD

CLAVICLE FRACTURE, OUTER THIRD, 1ST DEGREE

CLAVICLE FRACTURE, OUTER THIRD, 2ND DEGREE

Clavicle Fracture, Neer Type I: CLAVICLE FRACTURE, OUTER THIRD, 1ST DEGREE

Clavicle Fracture, Neer Type II: CLAVICLE FRACTURE, OUTER THIRD, 2ND DEGREE

Clavus Durum: CORN, HARD

Clavus Molle: CORN, SOFT

Cleat Laceration: LACERATION, SKIN

Cleat Puncture: WOUND, PENETRATING

Closed Fracture: FRACTURE, CLOSED (gl)

Clothesline Injury: LARYNX INJURY

COCCYGODYNIA

COCCYX FRACTURE

Cold, Common: RHINITIS, ACUTE

Collar Button Abscess: ABSCESS, COLLAR BUTTON

COLLES FRACTURE

Colles Fracture, Reversed: SMITH FRACTURE

Comminuted Fracture: FRACTURE, COMMINUTED (gl)

Complete Fracture: FRACTURE, COMPLETE (gl)

Compound Fracture: FRACTURE, OPEN (gl)

Compression Fracture: FRACTURE, COMPRESSION (gl)

Concussion, Abdominal: CELIAC PLEXUS SYNDROME

Concussion, Cauda Equina: CAUDA EQUINA CONCUSSION

Concussion, Cerebral: see CEREBRAL CONCUSSION, . . .

Concussion, Conus Medullaris: CONUS MEDULLARIS CONCUSSION

Concussion, Spinal Cord: SPINAL CORD CONCUSSION

CONFUSION (gl)

Conjunctivitis: EYE, CONJUNCTIVITIS, TRAUMATIC

CONTUSION

CONSCIOUSNESS (gl)

Conversion Reaction: ANXIETY REACTION

CONUS MEDULLARIS CONCUSSION

CONUS MEDULLARIS CONTUSION

CONVULSION (gl)

CORN, HARD

CORN, SOFT

Corporis Seborrhea: DERMATITIS, SEBORRHEIC

Cornea: see EYE, . . .

COSTOCHONDRAL SPRAIN

COSTOVERTEBRAL SPRAIN

COTTONMOUTH (gl)

134

Cotton's Fracture: ANKLE FRACTURE, ABDUCTION, 2ND DEGREE

Coxa Vara, Adolescent: FEMUR, SLIPPING PROXIMAL EPIPHYSIS

Crabs: PEDICULOSIS PUBIS

Cramp: MUSCLE CRAMP (gl)

CRANIOCEREBRAL HEMATOMA, EPIDURAL

CRANIOCEREBRAL HEMATOMA, SUBDURAL

Crazy Bone: FUNNY BONE (gl)

Cruciate Ligament Sprain: KNEE SPRAIN, ANTERIOR or POSTERIOR
   CRUCIATE LIGAMENT

Cryptorchidism: CRYPTORCHISM

CRYPTORCHISM

CUBOID FRACTURE

CUNEIFORM FRACTURE

Delayed Union Fracture: FRACTURE, DELAYED UNION (gl)

DELIRIUM, POST-TRAUMATIC (gl)

Deltoid Ligament Sprain: ANKLE SPRAIN, DELTOID LIGAMENT

deltoid, Sub-, Bursitis: SUBACROMIAL BURSITIS

DEMENTIA, POST-TRAUMATIC (gl)

DENTAL CARIES

Dentoalveolar Abscess: TOOTH ABSCESS

deQuervain's Disease: TENOSYNOVITIS, STENOSING

DERMATITIS, CONTACT

Dermatitis, External Ear: EAR, OTITIS EXTERNA, ACUTE

Dermatitis Medicamentosa: DRUG ERUPTIONS

dermatitis, Neuro-, Localized: NEURODERMATITIS, LOCALIZED

DERMATITIS, SEBORRHEIC

Dermatomycosis Furfuracea: TINEA VERSICOLOR

DERMATOPHYTID

Dermatophytosis: ATHLETE'S FOOT

Dhobie Itch: TINEA CRURIS

DIABETES MELLITUS

DIARRHEA (gl)

DISC RUPTURE, CERVICAL

DISC RUPTURE, LUMBAR

Displaced Fracture: FRACTURE, DISPLACED (gl)

DORSIFLEXION (gl)

DROWNING, FRESH WATER

drowning, Near-: NEAR-DROWNING (gl)

DRUG ERUPTIONS

DRYING OUT (gl)

DuPuytren's Fracture: ANKLE FRACTURE, ABDUCTION, 2ND
   DEGREE

135

Dysmenorrhea, Acquired: DYSMENORRHEA, SECONDARY

Dysmenorrhea, Essential: DYSMENORRHEA, PRIMARY

DYSMENORRHEA, PRIMARY

DYSMENORRHEA, SECONDARY

DYSPEPSIA (gl)

EAR, CAULIFLOWER

EAR DRUM, TRAUMATIC PERFORATION

Ear, Early Cauliflower: EAR, HEMATOMA, ACUTE

EAR, HEMATOMA, ACUTE

EAR, IMPACTED CERUMEN

EAR, OTITIS EXTERNA, ACUTE

EAR, OTITIS MEDIA, ACUTE

Ear, Swimmer's: EAR, OTITIS EXTERNA, ACUTE

Ear, Traumatic Deformity: EAR, CAULIFLOWER

ECCHYMOSIS (gl)

ELBOW DISLOCATION, ANTERIOR

ELBOW DISLOCATION, POSTERIOR

Elbow Fracture: ULNAR FRACTURE, OLECRANON

Elbow, Little League: HUMERUS FRACTURE, MEDIAL EPICONDYLE
EPIPHYSIS AVULSION

ELBOW OSTEOCHONDRITIS DISSECANS

Embolism, Fat: FAT EMBOLISM

Embolism, Pulmonary: PULMONARY EMBOLISM

ENDOMETRIOSIS

EPIDIDYMITIS, ACUTE

Epidural Cerebral Hematoma: CRANIOCEREBRAL HEMATOMA,
EPIDURAL

Epidural Spinal Hemorrhage: SPINAL HEMORRHAGE, EXTRADURAL

EPILEPSY, FOCAL

EPILEPSY, GRAND MAL

Epilepsy, Major: EPILEPSY, GRAND MAL

Epilepsy, Minor: EPILEPSY, PETIT MAL

EPILEPSY, JACKSONIAN

EPILEPSY, PETIT MAL

EPILEPSY, POST-TRAUMATIC

EILEPSY, PSYCHOMOTOR

Epilepsy, Pykno-: EPILEPSY, PETIT MAL

EPIPHYSEAL PLATE COMPRESSION FRACTURE

Epiphyseal Plate Injury, Type I: EPIPHYSEAL PLATE SEPARATION

Epiphyseal Plate Injury, Type II: EPIPHYSIS FRACTURE-SEPARATION,
1ST DEGREE

Epiphyseal Plate Injury, Type III: EPIPHYSIS FRACTURE-
SEPARATION, 2ND DEGREE

Epiphyseal Plate Injury, Type IV: EPIPHYSIS FRACTURE-
SEPARATION, 3RD DEGREE

Epipsyseal Plate Injury, Type V: EPIPHYSEAL PLATE COMPRESSION
FRACTURE

EPIPHYSEAL PLATE SEPARATION

EPIPHYSIS FRACTURE-SEPARATION, 1ST DEGREE

EPIPHYSIS FRACTURE-SEPARATION, 2ND DEGREE

EPIPHYSIS FRACTURE-SEPARATION, 3RD DEGREE

EPISTAXIS (gl)

ERYTHEMA (gl)

EVERSION (gl)

Exomphalos: HERNIA, UMBILICAL

Exostoses, Talotibial: ANKLE EXOSTOSES, TALOTIBIAL

EXOSTOSIS (gl)

EXTENSION (gl)

EXTENSOR DIGITORUS LONGUS TENOSYNOVITIS (TOE)

EXTENSOR HALLUCIS LONGUS TENOSYNOVITIS

Extradural Cerebral Hemorrhage: CRANIOCEREBRAL HEMATOMA,
EPIDURAL

Extradural Spinal Hemorrhage: SPINAL HEMORRHAGE,
EXTRADURAL

Extraoral Laceration: MOUTH, EXTRAORAL LACERATION

EYE, CONJUNCTIVITIS, TRAUMATIC

EYE, CORNEAL INJURY

EYE, CORNEAL OPACITY

EYE, CORNEAL ULCER

EYE, GLOBE INJURY

Eye, Hyphema: HYPHEMA (gl)

EYE, IRIS INJURY

EYE, PERIORBITAL HEMATOMA

EYE, RETINAL DETACHMENT

Eyeball Injury: EYE, GLOBE INJURY

FABELLA FRACTURE

Facets, Cervical, Overriding: SPINE DISLOCATION, CERVICAL
ARTICULAR PROCESS

Fascial Hernia: HERNIA, MUSCLE

FACE CONTUSION

FAT EMBOLISM

FAT PAD, INFRAPATELLAR, CONTUSION

Fat Pad Pinch: FAT PAD, INFRAPATELLAR, CONTUSION

Fatigue Fracture: FRACTURE, FATIGUE (gl)

FELON

Femur Fracture, Dicondylar: FEMUR FRACTURE, INTERCONDYLAR

Femur Fracture, Extracapsular: FEMUR FRACTURE, TROCHANTERIC

FEMUR FRACTURE, GREATER TROCHANTER

FEMUR FRACTURE, HEAD

FEMUR FRACTURE, INTERCONDYLAR

Femur Fracture, Intracapsular: FEMUR FRACTURE, NECK

FEMUR FRACTURE, LATERAL CONDYLE

FEMUR FRACTURE, LATERAL CONDYLE, CHONDRAL

FEMUR FRACTURE, LATERAL CONDYLE, OSTEOCHONDRAL

FEMUR FRACTURE, LESSER TROCHANTER

FEMUR FRACTURE, MEDIAL CONDYLE

FEMUR FRACTURE, MEDIAL CONDYLE, CHONDRAL

FEMUR FRACTURE, MEDIAL CONDYLE, OSTEOCHONDRAL

FEMUR FRACTURE, NECK

Femur Fracture, Neck, Basilar: FEMUR FRACTURE, TROCHANTERIC

FEMUR FRACTURE, POSTERIOR CONDYLE

FEMUR FRACTURE, SHAFT

FEMUR FRACTURE, SHAFT, FATIGUE

Femur Fracture, Subcapital: FEMUR FRACTURE, NECK

FEMUR FRACTURE, SUPRACONDYLAR

Femur Fracture, "T": FEMUR FRACTURE, INTERCONDYLAR

Femur Fracture, Transcervical: FEMUR FRACTURE, NECK

FEMUR FRACTURE, TROCHANTERIC

FEMUR FRACTURE-SEPARATION, DISTAL EPIPHYSIS

FEMUR FRACTURE-SEPARATION, PROXIMAL EPIPHYSIS

FEMUR OSTEOCHONDRITIS DISSECANS, LATERAL CONDYLE

FEMUR OSTEOCHONDRITIS DISSECANS, MEDIAL CONDYLE

FEMUR, SLIPPING PROXIMAL EPIPHYSIS

Fibula Dislocation, Upper End: SUPERIOR TIBIOFIBULAR
    DISLOCATION

Fibula Fracture, Distal End: ANKLE FRACTURE, EXTERNAL
    ROTATION

FIBULA FRACTURE, HEAD

Fibula Fracture, Lateral Malleolus: see ANKLE FRACTURE, . . .

FIBULA FRACTURE, NECK

FIBULA FRACTURE, SHAFT

FIBULA FRACTURE, SHAFT, FATIGUE

FIBULA FRACTURE, UPPER END

FIBULA FRACTURE-DISLOCATION, UPPER END

FIBULAR COLLATERAL LIGAMENT BURSITIS

Fibular Collateral Ligament Sprain, Ankle: ANKLE SPRAIN, FIBULAR
    COLLATERAL LIGAMENT

Fibular Collateral Ligament Sprain, Knee: KNEE SPRAIN, LATERAL
    COLLATERAL LIGAMENT

Fibular Head Bursitis: FIBULAR COLLATERAL BURSITIS
Finger, Baseball: BASEBALL FINGER
Finger, Cellulitis: FELON
FINGER DISLOCATION, INTERPHALANGEAL
FINGER FRACTURE, DISTAL PHALANX
FINGER FRACTURE, MIDDLE PHALANX
FINGER FRACTURE, PROXIMAL PHALANX
FINGER FRACTURE, "T" TYPE
Finger, Hammer: BASEBALL FINGER
Finger, Jammed: FINGER SPRAIN, PROXIMAL INTERPHALANGEAL
FINGER SPRAIN, PROXIMAL INTERPHALANGEAL
Finger, Stoved: FINGER SPRAIN, PROXIMAL INTERPHALANGEAL
Finger, Trigger: TENOSYNOVITIS, STENOSING
FLATFEET, SYMPTOMATIC
Flatfoot, Peroneal Spastic: PERONEAL SPASTIC FLATFOOT
FLEXION (gl)
FLEXOR DIGITORUM LONGUS TENOSYNOVITIS (TOE)
FLEXOR HALLUCIS LONGUS TENOSYNOVITIS
Floorburn: ABRASION
Flu: INFLUENZA
FOOD POISONING, STAPHYLOCOCCAL
FOOT CONTUSION, PLANTAR
Foot Ringworm: ATHLETE'S FOOT
FRACTURE (gl)
FRACTURE, ANGULATION (gl)
FRACTURE, AVULSION (gl)
FRACTURE, CHONDRAL (gl)
FRACTURE, CLOSED (gl)
FRACTURE, COMMINUTED (gl)
FRACTURE, COMPLETE (gl)
Fracture, Compound: FRACTURE, OPEN (gl)
FRACTURE, COMPRESSION (gl)
FRACTURE, DELAYED UNION (gl)
FRACTURE, DISPLACED (gl)
FRACTURE, FATIGUE (gl)
FRACTURE, GREENSTICK (gl)
FRACTURE, IMPACTED (gl)
FRACTURE, INCOMPLETE (gl)
FRACTURE, MALUNION (gl)
FRACTURE, NONUNION (gl)
FRACTURE, OBLIQUE (gl)
FRACTURE, OPEN (gl)

FRACTURE, OSTEOCHONDRAL (gl)

FRACTURE, OVERRIDING (gl)

FRACTURE, PATHOLOGICAL (gl)

FRACTURE, ROTATED (gl)

FRACTURE, SPIRAL (gl)

Fracture, Ununited: FRACTURE, NONUNION (gl)

FRACTURE-DISLOCATION (gl)

Fracture-Separation: see EPIPHYSIS, FRACTURE-SEPARATION

Freiberg's Disease: METATARSAL OSTEOCHONDRITIS, HEAD

FROSTBITE

FUNNY BONE (gl)

FURUNCULOSIS

GALEAZZI'S FRACTURE

GANGLION

GANGRENE (gl)

Gash: LACERATION, SKIN

Gastrocnemius Strain: CALF STRAIN

Gastrocnemius, Medial, Bursitis: POPLITEAL CYST

GASTROENTERITIS, ACUTE

Gaulding: INTERTRIGO

GENU RECURVATUM (gl)

GENU VALGUM (gl)

GINGIVITIS

Glandular Fever: MONONUCLEOSIS, INFECTIOUS

GLENOHUMERAL DISLOCATION, ANTERIOR

GLENOHUMERAL DISLOCATION, DOWNWARD

GLENOHUMERAL DISLOCATION, POSTERIOR

GLENOHUMERAL SUBLUXATION, ANTERIOR, RECURRENT

GLENOHUMERAL SUBLUXATION, POSTERIOR, RECURRENT

GLUTEUS MEDIUS STRAIN

GRACILIS STRAIN

GRANULOMA, SWIMMING POOL

Grassburn: ABRASION

Greenstick Fracture: FRACTURE, GREENSTICK (gl)

Grip: INFLUENZA

GROIN CONTUSION

Groin Ringworm: TINEA CRURIS

Groin Strain: ILIOPSOAS STRAIN

Hallux Malleus: TOE, HAMMER (gl)

HALLUX RIGIDUS (gl)

HALLUX VALGUS (gl)

Hammer Finger: BASEBALL FINGER

140

Hammer Toe: TOE, HAMMER (gl)

HAMSTRING STRAIN

HAMSTRING TENOSYNOVITIS

Hangman's Fracture: SPINE FRACTURE, HANGMAN'S

HAY FEVER

HEADACHE (gl)

HEART, AORTA COARCTATION

HEART, AORTIC VALVE STENOSIS, CONGENITAL

HEART, AORTIC VALVE STENOSIS, RHEUMATIC

Heart, Athlete's: ATHLETE'S HEART (gl)

Heart, Anomalous Atrioventricular Excitation: WOLFF-PARKINSON-
WHITE SYNDROME

Heart, Bradycardia: BRADYCARDIA (gl)

HEART BURN (gl)

HEART, INTERVENTRICULAR SEPTAL DEFECT

HEART, MITRAL VALVE INSUFFICIENCY

HEART, MITRAL VALVE STENOSIS

HEART MURMUR (gl)

HEART, MYOCARDIAL INFARCTION

HEART, MYOCARDIUM CONTUSION

HEART, PATENT DUCTUS ARTERIOSUS

HEART, PERICARDITIS, ACUTE

HEART, PULMONARY VALVE INSUFFICIENCY

HEART, PULMONARY VALVE STENOSIS

HEART, RHEUMATIC DISEASE, ACTIVE

Heart, Sinus, Arrhythmia: ARRHYTHMIA, SINUS (gl)

HEART, TACHYCARDIA, PAROXYSMAL ATRIAL

HEART, TACHYCARDIA, SINUS

HEAT EXHAUSTION

HEAT FATIGUE (gl)

Heat Prostration: HEAT EXHAUSTION

HEAT RASH

HEAT STROKE

Heat Syncope: HEAT EXHAUSTION

Heel Cord: see ACHILLES TENDON

Heloma Durum: CORN, HARD

Heloma Molle: CORN, SOFT

HEMARTHROSIS (gl)

HEMATOCELE, TUNICA VAGINALIS, TRAUMATIC

HEMATOMA (gl)

Hematomyelia, Spinal Cord: SPINAL CORD HEMATOMYELIA

HEMATURIA, MICROSCOPIC (gl)

HEMOPTYSIS (gl)

HEMORRHOIDS, THROMBOSED

HEPATITIS, INFECTIOUS

Hernia, Fascial: HERNIA, MUSCLE

HERNIA, INGUINAL, DIRECT

HERNIA, INGUINAL, INDIRECT

HERNIA, MUSCLE

Hernia, Synovial: GANGLION

HERNIA, UMBILICAL

HERPES SIMPLEX

Herpes Simplex Gladiatorum: HERPES SIMPLEX, TRAUMATIC

HERPES SIMPLEX, TRAUMATIC

Hip, Clicking: HIP, SNAPPING

HIP DISLOCATION, ANTERIOR

HIP DISLOCATION, POSTERIOR

HIP OSTEOCHONDRITIS DISSECANS

HIP POINTER

HIP, SNAPPING

HIP SPRAIN

HIP STRAIN

HIVES

Hoarseness: LARYNGITIS, ACUTE

Hordeolum, External: STY, EXTERNAL

HOT SPOT (gl)

Housemaid's Knee: PREPATELLAR BURSITIS

HUMERUS EPICONDYLITIS, LATERAL

HUMERUS EPICONDYLITIS, MEDIAL

HUMERUS FRACTURE, DICONDYLAR

Humerus Fracture, Distal, Transverse: HUMERUS FRACTURE,
    DICONDYLAR

Humerus Fracture, Epitrochlear: HUMERUS FRACTURE, MEDIAL
    EPICONDYLE

HUMERUS FRACTURE, GREATER TUBEROSITY

HUMERUS FRACTURE, LATERAL EPICONDYLE

HUMERUS FRACTURE, MEDIAL EPICONDYLE

HUMERUS FRACTURE, MEDIAL EPICONDYLE EPIPHYSIS
    AVULSION

HUMERUS FRACTURE, NECK, ABDUCTION

HUMERUS FRACTURE, NECK, ADDUCTION

HUMERUS FRACTURE, NECK EPIPHYSIS

HUMERUS FRACTURE, SHAFT

HUMERUS FRACTURE, SUPRACONDYLAR, EXTENSION

HUMERUS FRACTURE, SUPRACONDYLAR, FLEXION

HYDROCELE, TUNICA VAGINALIS

HYDROCELE, TUNICA VAGINALIS, TRAUMATIC

HYPERHIDROSIS

HYPERTENSION, LABILE (gl)

HYPERVENTILATION SYNDROME

HYPHEMA (gl)

HYPOGLYCEMIA (gl)

Hysteria Neurosis: ANXIETY REACTION

Iliac Crest Contusion: HIP POINTER

ILIOPECTINEAL BURSITIS

ILIOPSOAS STRAIN

ILIUM FRACTURE, CREST AVULSION

ILIUM FRACTURE, SPINE AVULSION

ILIUM FRACTURE, WING

Ilium Fracture-Separation, Crest Epiphysis: ILIUM FRACTURE, WING

Impacted Fracture: FRACTURE, IMPACTED (gl)

IMPETIGO

Impetigo Contagiosa: IMPETIGO

Incomplete Fracture: FRACTURE, INCOMPLETE (gl)

Infarction, Myocardial: HEART, MYOCARDIAL INFARCTION

Infarction, Pulmonary: PULMONARY EMBOLISM

Infectious Hepatitis: HEPATITIS, INFECTIOUS

Infectious Mononucleosis: MONONUCLEOSIS, INFECTIOUS

INFLUENZA

INFRAPATELLAR BURSITIS

Infrapatellar Fat Pad Contusion: FAT FAD, INFRAPATELLAR,
    CONTUSION

Infraspinatus Strain: ROTATOR CUFF STRAIN, . . .

Ingrown Toenail: NAIL, TOE, INGROWN

Inguinal Hernia: HERNIA, INGUINAL, DIRECT or INDIRECT

INTERNAL CAROTID ARTERY OCCLUSION

Interphalangeal Dislocation, Finger: FINGER DISLOCATION,
    INTERPHALANGEAL

Interphalangeal Dislocation, Toe: TOE DISLOCATION,
    INTERPHALANGEAL

Interphalangeal Sprain, Finger: FINGER SPRAIN, PROXIMAL
    INTERPHALANGEAL

INTERTRIGO

INTRACEREBRAL HEMORRHAGE

Intramedullary Spinal Hemorrhage: SPINAL CORD HEMATOMYELIA

Intraoral Laceration: MOUTH, INTRAORAL LACERATION

INVERSION (gl)

Iris Injury: EYE, IRIS INJURY
Ischial Tuberosity Bursitis: ISCHIOGLUTEAL BURSITIS
ISCHIOGLUTEAL BURSITIS
ISCHIOPUBIC FRACTURE, RAMI
ISCHIOPUBIC FRACTURE, RAMI AVULSION
ISCHIUM FRACTURE, INFERIOR RAMUS
ISCHIUM FRACTURE, SUPERIOR RAMUS
ISCHIUM FRACTURE, TUBEROSITY
ISCHIUM FRACTURE, TUBEROSITY AVULSION
Jammed Finger: FINGER SPRAIN, PROXIMAL INTERPHALANGEAL
Jammed Neck: CERVICAL SPINE SPRAIN
Jaundice, Yellow: HEPATITIS, INFECTIOUS
Jaw Dislocation: TEMPOROMANDIBULAR DISLOCATION
Jaw Fracture (Lower): MANDIBLE FRACTURE
Jock Itch: TINEA CRURIS
JOINT DISLOCATION
JOINT LOOSE BODIES
Joint Luxation: JOINT DISLOCATION
Joint Mice: JOINT LOOSE BODIES
JOINT SUBLUXATION
KIDNEY CONTUSION
KIDNEY LACERATION
Knee, Anserine Bursitis: ANSERINE BURSITIS
KNEE CALCIFICATION, MEDIAL COLLATERAL LIGAMENT
KNEE CONTUSION
KNEE DISLOCATION
Knee, Housemaid's: PREPATELLAR BURSITIS
KNEE, INTERNAL DERANGEMENT (gl)
Knee Ossification, Post-traumatic Para-articular: KNEE CALCIFICATION,
    MEDIAL COLLATERAL LIGAMENT
KNEE ROTARY INSTABILITY (gl)
KNEE SPRAIN, ANTERIOR CRUCIATE LIGAMENT
KNEE SPRAIN, HYPEREXTENSION
KNEE SPRAIN, LATERAL COLLATERAL LIGAMENT
KNEE SPRAIN, MEDIAL COLLATERAL LIGAMENT
Knee Sprain, Medial Capsule: KNEE ROTARY INSTABILITY (gl)
KNEE SPRAIN, POSTERIOR CRUCIATE LIGAMENT
Knock Knee: GENU VALGUM (gl)
Koehler II Disease: METATARSAL HEAD OSTEOCHONDRITIS
Kyphosis, Juvenile: VERTEBRAL EPIPHYSITIS, DORSAL
LACE BITE (gl)
LACERATION, SKIN

Larsen-Johansson's Disease: PATELLA OSTEOCHONDRITIS

LARYNGITIS, ACUTE

LARYNX INJURY

Lateral Collateral Ligament Sprain, Ankle: ANKLE SPRAIN, FIBULAR COLLATERAL LIGAMENT

Lateral Collateral Ligament Sprain, Knee: KNEE SPRAIN, LATERAL COLLATERAL LIGAMENT

Lichen Simplex, Chronic: NEURODERMATITIS, LOCALIZED

Lime Burn: BURN, CHEMICAL

Little League Elbow: HUMERUS FRACTURE, MEDIAL EPICONDYLE EPIPHYSIS AVULSION

Low Back Pain: LUMBOSACRAL SPRAIN

Lumbago: LUMBOSACRAL STRAIN

Lumbar Arthritis, Traumatic: SPONDYLOSIS, LUMBAR

Lumbar Disc Rupture: DISC RUPTURE, LUMBAR

Lumbar Spondylolisthesis: SPONDYLOLISTHESIS, LUMBAR

Lumbar Spondylolysis: SPONDYLOLYSIS, LUMBAR

Lumbar Spondylosis: SPONDYLOSIS, LUMBAR

LUMBOSACRAL SPRAIN

LUMBOSACRAL STRAIN

lunar, Peri-, Dislocation: PERILUNAR DISLOCATION

LUNATE DISLOCATION

Lung Collapse: PNEUMOTHORAX, SPONTANEOUS or TRAUMATIC

LYMPHADENITIS, ACUTE

LYMPHANGITIS, ACUTE

Malar Fracture: ZYGOMA FRACTURE

Mallet Finger: BASEBALL FINGER

Malunion Fracture: FRACTURE, MALUNION (gl)

MANDIBLE FRACTURE

March Fracture: FRACTURE, FATIGUE (gl)

Matburn: ABRASION

MAXILLA FRACTURE

MEDIAL COLLATERAL LIGAMENT BURSITIS (KNEE)

Medial Collateral Ligament Sprain, Ankle: ANKLE SPRAIN, DELTOID LIGAMENT

Medial Collateral Ligament Sprain, Knee: KNEE SPRAIN, MEDIAL COLLATERAL LIGAMENT

MEDIAL COLLATERAL LIGAMENT SYNDROME (KNEE)

MENISCUS, LATERAL, CYST

MENISCUS, LATERAL, DISCOID

MENISCUS, LATERAL, TEAR

MENISCUS, MEDIAL, CYST

MENISCUS, MEDIAL, TEAR

MENORRHAGIA (gl)

METACARPAL, FIRST, FRACTURE

Metacarpal, First, Fracture-Dislocation: BENNETT'S FRACTURE

METACARPAL FRACTURE, BASE

METACARPAL FRACTURE, NECK

METACARPAL FRACTURE, SHAFT

Metacarpal Fracture, Subcapital: METACARPAL FRACTURE, NECK

METACARPOPHALANGEAL DISLOCATION

METACARPOPHALANGEAL, FIRST, DISLOCATION

METACARPOPHALANGEAL, INDEX, VOLAR DISLOCATION

METACARPOPHALANGEAL SPRAIN

METATARSAL, FIFTH, FRACTURE, BASE

METATARSAL FRACTURE, BASE

METATARSAL FRACTURE, HEAD

METATARSAL FRACTURE, HEAD, CHONDRAL

METATARSAL FRACTURE, HEAD, OSTEOCHONDRAL

METATARSAL FRACTURE, NECK

METATARSAL FRACTURE, SHAFT

METATARSAL FRACTURE, SHAFT, FATIGUE

METATARSAL HEAD OSTEOCHONDRITIS

Metatarsalgia, Morton's: PLANTAR NEUROMA

METATARSOPHALANGEAL DISLOCATION

METRORRHAGIA (gl)

MIDTARSAL DISLOCATION

Miliaria Rubra: HEAT RASH

Mitral Valve: see HEART, . . .

Mittelschmertz: OVARIAN HEMORRHAGE

MOLLUSCUM CONTAGIOSUM

Molluscum Epitheliale: MOLLUSCUM CONTAGIOSUM

MONILIASIS, CUTANEOUS

MONONUCLEOSIS, INFECTIOUS

MONTEGGIA FRACTURE

Morton's Toe: PLANTAR NEUROMA

Mouse: PERIORBITAL HEMATOMA

MOUTH, EXTRAORAL LACERATION

MOUTH, INTRAORAL LACERATION

MUSCLE ATROPHY (gl)

MUSCLE CRAMP (gl)

Muscle Hernia: HERNIA, MUSCLE

Muscle Pull: See STRAIN, . . .

MYOPIA (gl)

MYOSITIS OSSIFICANS, TRAUMATIC

NAIL AVULSION

NAIL, SUBUNGUAL HEMATOMA

NAIL, TOE, INGROWN

NAUSEA (gl)

NEAR-DROWNING (gl)

Nearsightedness: MYOPIA (gl)

Neck Sprain: CERVICAL SPINE SPRAIN

Neer Type I Clavicle Fracture: CLAVICLE FRACTURE, OUTER
  THIRD, 1ST DEGREE

Neer Type II Clavicle Fracture: CLAVICLE FRACTURE, OUTER
  THIRD, 2ND DEGREE

Nerve Compression: NERVE CONTUSION

Nerve Inflammation: NEURITIS

Nerve Pinch: PINCHED NERVE SYNDROME (gl)

NEURITIS

Neuritis, Traumatic: NERVE CONTUSION

NEURODERMATITIS, LOCALIZED

Nonunion Fracture: FRACTURE, NONUNION (gl)

Nose Bleed: EPISTAXIS (gl)

NOSE CONTUSION

NOSE FRACTURE

Oblique Fracture: FRACTURE, OBLIQUE (gl)

OLECRANON BURSITIS

Open Fracture: FRACTURE, OPEN (gl)

ORBIT BLOWOUT FRACTURE

ORCHITIS, TRAUMATIC

Os Calcis: see CALCANEUS, . . .

OSGOOD-SCHLATTER'S DISEASE

OSTEOARTHRITIS (gl)

Osteochondral Fracture: FRACTURE, OSTEOCHONDRAL (gl)

OSTEOCHONDRITIS DISSECANS

OSTEOCHONDROMA

OSTEOCHONDROMATOSIS, SYNOVIAL

Osteoclastoma: BONE TUMOR, GIANT CELL

OSTEOGENIC SARCOMA

OSTEOID OSTEOMA

OSTEOMYELITIS, ACUTE

Otitis Externa, Acute: EAR, OTITIS EXTERNA, ACUTE

Otitis Media, Acute: EAR, OTITIS MEDIA, ACUTE

OVARIAN HEMORRHAGE

Overriding Fracture: FRACTURE OVERRIDING (gl)

Palmar Space Abscess: ABSCESS, PALMAR SPACE

PARAPLEGIA (gl)

PARONYCHIA

PATELLA BIPARTITE (gl)

PATELLA CHONDROMALACIA

PATELLA DISLOCATION, ACUTE

PATELLA DISLOCATION, RECURRENT

PATELLA FRACTURE

PATELLA FRACTURE, AVULSION, INFERIOR POLE

PATELLA FRACTURE, AVULSION, SUPERIOR POLE

PATELLA FRACTURE, CHONDRAL

PATELLA FRACTURE, LATERAL MARGINAL

PATELLA FRACTURE, MEDIAL TANGENTIAL

PATELLA FRACTURE, OSTEOCHONDRAL

PATELLA OSTEOCHONDRITIS

PATELLA OSTEOCHONDRITIS DISSECANS

PATELLA SUBLUXATION, ACUTE

PATELLA SUBLUXATION, RECURRENT

PATELLAR TENDON STRAIN

patellar, Infra-, Bursitis: INFRAPATELLAR BURSITIS

patellar, Infra-, Fat Pad Contusion: FAT PAD, INFRAPATELLAR, CONTUSION

patellar, Pre-, Bursitis: PREPATELLAR BURSITIS

Patellar Tubercle Avulsion Fracture: TIBIA FRACTURE, TUBERCLE AVULSION

Patent Ductus Arteriosus: HEART, PATENT DUCTUS ARTERIOSUS

Pathological Fracture: FRACTURE, PATHOLOGICAL (gl)

PEDICULOSIS PUBIS

Pellegrini-Stieda Disease: KNEE CALCIFICATION, MEDIAL COLLATERAL LIGAMENT

Pelvic Endometriosis: ENDOMETRIOSIS

PELVIS FRACTURE

PEPTIC ULCER SYNDROME

Periapical Abscess: TOOTH ABSCESS

Pericarditis: HEART, PERICARDITIS

PERILUNAR DISLOCATION

PERIODONTITIS

PERIOSTITIS, TRAUMATIC

PERONEAL NERVE CONTUSION

PERONEAL SPASTIC FLATFOOT

PERONEAL TENDON DISLOCATION, ACUTE
PERONEAL TENDON DISLOCATION, RECURRENT
PERONEAL TENDON TENOSYNOVITIS
PES CAVUS (gl)
PHARYNGITIS, ACUTE
Phlegmon: CELLULITIS
Piedmont Fracture: GALEAZZI FRACTURE
Piles: HEMORRHOIDS, THROMBOSED
PILONIDAL CYST
Pimples: ACNE VULGARIS
PINCHED NERVE SYNDROME (gl)
Pityriasis Versicolor: TINEA VERSICOLOR
PITYRIASIS ROSEA
Plantar Contusion: FOOT CONTUSION, PLANTAR
PLANTAR FASCIITIS
PLANTARFLEXION (gl)
PLANTAR NEUROMA
PLANTAR WART
PLANTARIS STRAIN
PNEUMONIA, ACUTE
PNEUMOTHORAX, SPONTANEOUS
PNEUMOTHORAX, TRAUMATIC
Pollenosis: HAY FEVER
Popliteal Bursitis: POPLITEAL CYST
POPLITEAL CYST
POPLITEUS TENDON AVULSION
POST-CONCUSSION SYNDRONE (gl)
POSTERIOR TIBIAL TENDON DISLOCATION
POSTERIOR TIBIAL TENDON TENOSYNOVITIS
Pott's Fracture: ANKLE FRACTURE, ABDUCTION, 2ND DEGREE
Prehallux Fracture: ACCESSORY TARSAL NAVICULAR FRACTURE
PREPATELLAR BURSITIS
Prickly Heat Rash: HEAT RASH
Prizefighter's Ear: EAR, CAULIFLOWER
PRONATION (gl)
PROSTATITIS
PRURITUS, ANI (gl)
PUBIC SYMPHYSIS DISLOCATION
PUBIS FRACTURE, INFERIOR RAMUS
PUBIS FRACTURE, SUPERIOR RAMUS

PULMONARY EMBOLISM

Pulmonary Valve: see HEART, . . .

Punch Drunk Syndrome: BRAIN SYNDROME, CHRONIC

Puncture Wound: WOUND, PENETRATING

Purulent Arthritis: ARTHRITIS, SUPPURATIVE

Pyarthrosis: ARTHRITIS, SUPPURATIVE

PYELONEPHRITIS, ACUTE

Pyogenic Arthritis: ARTHRITIS, SUPPURATIVE

Pyorrhea: PERIODONTITIS

Quadriceps Contusion: CHARLEYHORSE

QUADRICEPS STRAIN

QUADRICEPS TENDON STRAIN

Quadriplegia: TETRAPLEGIA (gl)

Radiohumeral Bursitis: HUMERUS EPICONDYLITIS, LATERAL

RADIOULNAR DISLOCATION, INFERIOR

RADIOULNAR FRACTURE

RADIUS DISLOCATION, HEAD

Radius Fracture, Distal End: see BARTON, COLLES, GALEAZZI, and
    SMITH FRACTURES

RADIUS FRACTURE, DISTAL EPIPHYSIS

RADIUS FRACTURE, HEAD-NECK

RADIUS FRACTURE, SHAFT

RECTUS FEMORIS STRAIN

Retina, Detached: EYE, RETINAL DETACHMENT

Retrocalcaneal Bursitis: ACHILLOBURSITIS

Retrolunar Dislocation: PERILUNAR DISLOCATION

RHEUMATIC FEVER, ACUTE

Rheumatic Heart Disease: HEART, RHEUMATIC DISEASE, ACTIVE

Rheumatoid Spondylitis: SPONDYLITIS, RHEUMATOID

RHINITIS, ACUTE

Rhinitis, Allergic: HAY FEVER

Rib-Cartilage Injury: COSTOCHONDRAL SPRAIN

RIB FRACTURE

Ringworm, Foot: ATHLETE'S FOOT

Ringworm, Groin: TINEA CRURIS

Rotated Fracture: FRACTURE, ROTATED (gl)

ROTATOR CUFF STRAIN, 1ST DEGREE

ROTATOR CUFF STRAIN, 2ND DEGREE

ROTATOR CUFF STRAIN, 3RD DEGREE

Roundback, Adolescent: VERTEBRAL EPIPHYSITIS, DORSAL

SACROCOCCYGEAL DISLOCATION

SACROILIAC DISLOCATION

SACRUM FRACTURE

Sarcoma, Osteogenic: OSTEOGENIC SARCOMA

SARTORIUS STRAIN

Scaphoid Fracture: CARPAL NAVICULAR FRACTURE

SCAPULA FRACTURE

Scapulohumeral Bursitis: SUBACROMIAL BURSITIS

Scheuermann's Disease: VERTEBRAL EPIPHYSITIS, DORSAL

Schneider's Syndrome: SPINAL CORD SYNDROME, ACUTE, CENTRAL CERVICAL

SCOLIOSIS

Scrape: ABRASION

SEBACEOUS CYST, INFECTED

Seborrheic Eczema: DERMATITIS, SEBORRHEIC

Semilunar Cartilage: see MENISCUS, . . .

Separation, Shoulder: ACROMIOCLAVICULAR SPRAIN, 2ND DEGREE

Septal Defect: HEART, INTERVENTRICULAR SEPTAL DEFECT

Septic Arthritis: ARTHRITIS, SUPPURATIVE

SEPTICEMIA (gl)

SEPTUM, DEVIATED (gl)

Sesamoid Fracture: TOE, GREAT, FRACTURE, SESAMOIDS

Sesamoiditis: TOE, GREAT, SESAMOIDITIS

Sever's Disease: CALCANEAL APOPHYSITIS

SHIN CONTUSION

SHIN SPLINTS (gl)

Shiner: PERIORBITAL HEMATOMA

SHOCK (gl)

Shoulder Dislocation: GLENOHUMERAL DISLOCATION, . . .

Shoulder Separation: see ACROMIOCLAVICULAR SPRAIN, . . .

Shoulder Subluxation: GLENOHUMERAL SUBLUXATION, . . .

SINUS TARSI SYNDROME

SINUSITIS

Skidburn: ABRASION

Skin Laceration: LACERATION, SKIN

SKULL FRACTURE

Slideburn: ABRASION

SMITH FRACTURE

Solar Plexus Syndrome: CELIAC PLEXUS SYNDROME

SPEARING (gl)

SPERMATIC CORD TORSION

SPINA BIFIDA OCCULTA

Spinal Arthritis, Atrophic: SPONDYLITIS, RHEUMATOID

Spinal Arthritis, Traumatic: SPONDYLOSIS, CERVICAL or LUMBAR

SPINAL CORD CONCUSSION

SPINAL CORD CONTUSION

SPINAL CORD HEMATOMYELIA

SPINAL CORD SYNDROME, ACUTE, ANTERIOR CERVICAL

SPINAL CORD SYNDROME, ACUTE, CENTRAL CERVICAL

SPINAL HEMORRHAGE, EXTRADURAL

Spinal Hemorrhage, Intramedullary: SPINAL CORD HEMATOMYELIA

SPINAL HEMORRHAGE, SUBDURAL

SPINE DISLOCATION, ATLANTOAXIAL

SPINE DISLOCATION, CERVICAL ARTICULAR PROCESS

SPINE FRACTURE, COMPRESSION

SPINE FRACTURE, HANGMAN'S

SPINE FRACTURE, SPINOUS PROCESS

SPINE FRACTURE, TEARDROP

SPINE FRACTURE, TRANSVERSE PROCESS

SPINE FRACTURE-DISLOCATION

Spine Sprain, Cervical: CERVICAL SPINE SPRAIN

Spine Sprain, Lumbar: LUMBOSACRAL SPRAIN

Spine Subluxation: SPINE FRACTURE-DISLOCATION

Spiral Fracture: FRACTURE, SPIRAL (gl)

SPLEEN CONTUSION

SPLEEN RUPTURE

Spondylitis, Ankylosing: SPONDYLITIS, RHEUMATOID

SPONDYLITIS, RHEUMATOID

SPONDYLOLISTHESIS, LUMBAR

SPONDYLOLYSIS, LUMBAR

SPONDYLOSIS, CERVICAL

SPONDYLOSIS, LUMBAR

SPRAIN, 1ST DEGREE

SPRAIN, 2ND DEGREE

SPRAIN, 3RD DEGREE

Sprain, Mild: SPRAIN, 1ST DEGREE

Sprain, Moderate: SPRAIN, 2ND DEGREE

Sprain, Severe: SPRAIN, 3RD DEGREE

Spur, Ankle: ANKLE EXOSTOSES, TALOTIBIAL

Spur, Heel: see PLANTAR FASCIITIS

STALE (gl)

Sternoclavicular Dislocation: STERNOCLAVICULAR SPRAIN, 3RD
   DEGREE

STERNOCLAVICULAR SPRAIN, 1ST DEGREE

STERNOCLAVICULAR SPRAIN, 2ND DEGREE

STERNOCLAVICULAR SPRAIN, 3RD DEGREE

Sternoclavicular Subluxation: STERNOCLAVICULAR SPRAIN, 2ND DEGREE

STERNUM FRACTURE

STING, INSECT

STITCH IN SIDE

Stone Bruise: FOOT CONTUSION, PLANTAR; or, PERIOSTITIS, TRAUMATIC

Stoved Finger: FINGER SPRAIN, PROXIMAL INTERPHALANGEAL

STRAIN, 1ST DEGREE

STRAIN, 2ND DEGREE

STRAIN, 3RD DEGREE

Strain, Mild: STRAIN, 1ST DEGREE

Strain, Moderate: STRAIN, 2ND DEGREE

Strain, Severe: STRAIN, 3RD DEGREE

Strawberry: ABRASION

Stress Fracture: FRACTURE, FATIGUE (gl)

stroke, Sun-: HEAT STROKE

Strumpell-Marie Disease: SPONDYLITIS, RHEUMATOID

STY, EXTERNAL

SUBACROMIAL BURSITIS

Subarachnoid Hemorrhage: CEREBRAL HEMORRHAGE, SUBARACHNOID

Subcoracoid Dislocation: GLENOHUMERAL DISLOCATION, ANTERIOR

Subdeltoid Bursitis: SUBACROMIAL BURSITIS

Subdural Hemorrhage: CRANIOCEREBRAL HEMATOMA, SUBDURAL

Subdural Hydroma, Hygroma: CEREBRAL HYDROMA, SUBDURAL

Subdural Spinal Hemorrhage: SPINAL HEMORRHAGE, SUBDURAL

Subglenoid Dislocation: GLENOHUMERAL DISLOCATION, DOWNWARD

SUBTALAR TALONAVICULAR DISLOCATION

Subungual Hematoma: NAIL, SUBUNGUAL HEMATOMA

Sugar Diabetes: DIABETES MELLITUS

Sun stroke: HEAT STROKE

SUPERIOR TIBIOFIBULAR DISLOCATION

SUPINATION (gl)

Supramalleolar Fracture: ANKLE FRACTURE, ABDUCTION, 3RD DEGREE

Supraspinatus Strain: ROTATOR CUFF STRAIN, . . .

Sweating, Excessive: HYPERHIDROSIS

Swimmer's Ear: EAR, OTITIS EXTERNA, ACUTE

Swimming Pool Granuloma: GRANULOMA, SWIMMING POOL

SYNCOPE (gl)

Synovial Hernia: GANGLION

Synovial Osteochondromatosis: OSTEOCHONDROMATOSIS, SYNOVIAL

SYNOVITIS, TRAUMATIC (gl)

Tachycardia: HEART, TACHYCARDIA

Tailbone Fracture: COCCYX FRACTURE

talar navicular, Sub-, Dislocation: SUBTALAR NAVICULAR DISLOCATION

Talotibial Exostoses: ANKLE EXOSTOSES, TALOTIBIAL

TALUS DISLOCATION

Talus Dome, Osteochondritis Dissecans: TALUS FRACTURE, DOME, OSTEOCHONDRAL

Talus Dome, Flake Fracture: TALUS FRACTURE, DOME, OSTEOCHONDRAL

TALUS FRACTURE, BODY

TALUS FRACTURE, DOME, OSTEOCHONDRAL, SUPEROLATERAL MARGIN

TALUS FRACTURE, DOME, OSTEOCHONDRAL, SUPEROMEDIAL MARGIN

TALUS FRACTURE, HEAD

TALUS FRACTURE, HEAD, AVULSION

TALUS FRACTURE, NECK

TALUS FRACTURE, POSTERIOR PROCESS

TALUS FRACTURE, POSTERIOR PROCESS AVULSION

TAPE BURN (gl)

tarsal, Mid-, Dislocation: MIDTARSAL DISLOCATION

TARSAL TUNNEL SYNDROME

TARSAL NAVICULAR FRACTURE

Tarsal Navicular Accessory Fracture: ACCESSORY TARSAL NAVICULAR FRACTURE

TARSAL NAVICULAR FRACTURE, AVULSION

TARSAL NAVICULAR FRACTURE, OSTEOCHONDRAL

Tarsal Scaphoid Fracture: TARSAL NAVICULAR FRACTURE

TARSOMETATARSAL DISLOCATION

Teardrop Fracture: SPINAL FRACTURE, TEARDROP

TEMPOROMANDIBULAR DISLOCATION

TENDINITIS

TENDON DISLOCATION (gl)

TENOSYNOVITIS

TENOSYNOVITIS, STENOSING

Teres Minor Strain: ROTATOR CUFF STRAIN, . . .

154

TESTIS INJURY

Testis, Undescended: CRYPTORCHISM

TETANUS

TETRAPLEGIA (gl)

THROMBOPHLEBITIS

Thumb Dislocation: CARPOMETACARPAL, FIRST, DISLOCATION

Thumb Fracture: METACARPAL, FIRST, FRACTURE

TIBIA FRACTURE, LATERAL CONDYLE

TIBIA FRACTURE, LATERAL CONDYLE AVULSION

TIBIA FRACTURE, MEDIAL CONDYLE

TIBIA FRACTURE, MEDIAL CONDYLE AVULSION

Tibia Fracture, Medial Malleolus: see ANKLE FRACTURE, . . .

TIBIA FRACTURE, POSTERIOR RIM AVULSION

TIBIA FRACTURE, SHAFT

TIBIA FRACTURE, SHAFT, FATIGUE

TIBIA FRACTURE, SPINE

TIBIA FRACTURE, TUBERCLE AVULSION

TIBIA FRACTURE, UPPER END

Tibia Fracture-Separation, Distal Epiphysis: ANKLE FRACTURE, EXTERNAL ROTATION, 3RD DEGREE

TIBIA FRACTURE-SEPARATION, UPPER EPIPHYSIS

Tibial Collateral Ligament: see Medial Collateral Ligament

Tibial Compartment Syndrome, Anterior: ANTERIOR TIBIAL COMPARTMENT SYNDROME

TIBIAL CONDYLE OSTEOCHONDRITIS DISSECANS

Tibial Exostosis: ANKLE EXOSTOSES, TALOTIBIAL

Tibial Tendon Tenosynovitis: see ANTERIOR or POSTERIOR TIBIAL TENDON TENOSYNOVITIS

Tibial Tubercle Osteochondritis: OSGOOD-SCHLATTER'S DISEASE

Tibiofemoral Dislocation: KNEE DISLOCATION

Tibiofibular Dislocation, Superior: SUPERIOR TIBIOFIBULAR DISLOCATION

Tibiofibular Fracture-Separation, Distal Epiphysis: ANKLE FRACTURE-SEPARATION, DISTAL TIBIOFIBULAR EPIPHYSIS

TINEA CRURIS

Tinea Pedis: ATHLETE'S FOOT

TINEA VERSICOLOR

TINNITUS (gl)

TOE DISLOCATION, INTERPHALANGEAL

TOE FRACTURE, AVULSION

TOE FRACTURE, PROXIMAL PHALANX

TOE FRACTURE, TIP TUFT

TOE, GREAT, DISLOCATION, INTERPHALANGEAL

TOE, GREAT, DISLOCATION, METATARSOPHALANGEAL

TOE, GREAT, FRACTURE, AVULSION

TOE, GREAT, FRACTURE, OSTEOCHONDRAL

TOE, GREAT, FRACTURE, PHALANX

TOE, GREAT, FRACTURE, SESAMOIDS

TOE, GREAT, SESAMOIDITIS

Toe, Great, Tenosynovitis: EXTENSOR or FLEXOR HALLUCIS LONGUS TENOSYNOVITIS

Toe, Hallux Rigidus: HALLUX RIGIDUS (gl)

Toe, Hallux Valgus: HALLUX VALGUS (gl)

TOE, HAMMER (gl)

Toe, Morton's: PLANTAR NEUROMA

Toe, Tenosynovitis: EXTENSOR or FLEXOR DIGITORUM LONGUS TENOSYNOVITIS (TOE)

Toenail, Ingrown: NAIL, TOE, INGROWN

TONSILLITIS, ACUTE

TOOTH ABSCESS

Tooth Caries: DENTAL CARIES

TOOTH EXTRUSION (gl)

TOOTH FRACTURE, BREAK

TOOTH FRACTURE, CHIP

TOOTH FRACTURE, LINEAR

TOOTH FRACTURE, ROOT

TOOTH, INTRUDED

TOOTH, LUXATED, COMPLETE

TOOTH, LUXATED, PARTIAL

Traumatic Arthritis: ARTHRITIS, TRAUMATIC

TRIAD, UNHAPPY (gl)

Trigger Finger: TENOSYNOVITIS, STENOSING

TRIGGER POINT (gl)

Trimalleolar Fracture: ANKLE FRACTURE, ABDUCTION, 2ND DEGREE

TROCHANTERIC BURSITIS

TUBERCULOSIS, PULMONARY

Tunica Vaginalis Hematocele: HEMATOCELE, TUNICA VAGINALIS

Tunica Vaginalis Hydrocele: HYDROCELE, TUNICA VAGINALIS

Ulcer: PEPTIC ULCER SYNDROME

ULNA FRACTURE, CENTRAL THIRD

ULNA FRACTURE, DISTAL THIRD

ULNA FRACTURE, OLECRANON

ULNA FRACTURE, PROXIMAL THIRD

Ulna Fracture, Shaft: MONTEGGIA FRACTURE

ULNAR NERVE DISLOCATION, RECURRENT

Umbilical Hernia: HERNIA, UMBILICAL

UNCONSCIOUSNESS (gl)

Unguinus Incarnatus: NAIL, TOE, INGROWN

Ununited Fracture: FRACTURE, NONUNION (gl)

Urticaria, Allergic: HIVES

Urticaria, Giant: ANGIONEUROTIC EDEMA

URTICARIA, NONALLERGENIC

VAGINITIS

VARICOCELE

VARICOSE VEINS (gl)

Venenata, Dermatitis: DERMATITIS, CONTACT

Verruca: WART

Verruca, Plantar: PLANTAR WART

VERTEBRA, TRANSITIONAL

VERTEBRAL ARTERY OCCLUSION

VERTEBRAL EPIPHYSITIS, DORSAL

Vertebral Fracture: see SPINE FRACTURE, . . .

Vertebral Osteochondritis: VERTEBRAL EPIPHYSITIS, DORSAL

VOLAR FLEXION (gl)

Volkmann's Ischemia of Leg: ANTERIOR TIBIAL COMPARTMENT
  SYNDROME

WART

Wart, Plantar: PLANTAR WART

Wart, Water: MOLLUSCUM, CONTAGIOSUM

Wax in Ear: EAR, IMPACTED CERUMEN

Web-Space Abscess: ABSCESS, PALMAR SPACE

Wen, Infected: SEBACEOUS CYST, INFECTED

WHIPLASH (gl)

WOLFF-PARKINSON-WHITE SYNDROME

Wound, Cleat, Lacerating: LACERATION, SKIN

Wound, Cleat, Puncture: WOUND, PENETRATING

WOUND, HUMAN BITE

Wound, Lacerating: LACERATION, SKIN

WOUND, PENETRATING

Wound, Puncture: WOUND, PENETRATING

Wrestler's Ear: EAR, CAULIFLOWER

WRIST SPRAIN, HYPEREXTENSION

WRIST SPRAIN, HYPERFLEXION

ZYGOMA FRACTURE

ZYGOMATIC ARCH FRACTURE